ARTHRITIS
The Natural Remedy

JOHN ROWLAND

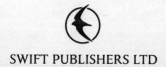

SWIFT PUBLISHERS LTD

© 1993 by John Rowland

Swift Publishers Ltd
Refuge Assurance House, Market Street, Bromsgrove,
Worcestershire, B61 8DA, England.

Swift Publishers Ltd, England
A subsidiary of Swift Consolidated Holdings PLC

British Library Cataloguing-in-Publication Data

Rowland, John
Arthritis – the Natural Remedy
I. World – Medical Self Help
II. Title
ISBN 1 874082 10 3

First published in Great Britain by Swift Publishers 1993

Designed & typeset in Columbus by Armitage Typo/Graphics
Riverside Studios, Dogley Mill, Fenay Bridge, Huddersfield HD8 OLE

Printed and bound in the UK by Harper Collins, Wester Hill Road, Bishopbriggs, Glasgow G20

To
Beulah
Mark James
Olive and Pop

Acknowledgements

I would like to thank my colleagues, family and friends for their help in compiling this book, in particular Angus Thomas, BSC, CCheM, FRSC, Christopher Thompson MIBiol, GRIB, AIB, ASAB, Valerie Bird and the late Alice and Harry Pollard.

Letters to the author will be most welcome and should be addressed to:
Mr John Rowland
Consultant Herbalist
The Naturopathic Private Clinic
76 Victoria Road East
Thornton, Lancashire FY5 5HH

Contents

Introduction

By Dr Frank Ryan, consultant physician and co-author of *The Eskimo Diet*.

In the UK alone, arthritis in its various forms afflicts an astonishing twenty million people, taking the joy out of life and condemning those more seriously affected to an existence of pain and disability. It is usually thought of as a disease of the elderly, but although the risk of developing some types of arthritis increases with age, by and large it is no respecter of age, sex, race or social status: perhaps one of the saddest statistics is the fact that 15,000 of these sufferers are children with rheumatoid arthritis.

For a very long time, we in the medical profession have been trying to find a cure. But although we understand the causative mechanisms of certain forms, such as gout, the root cause or causes of the most common forms of arthritis, rheumatoid arthritis and osteoarthritis, have evaded our most intensive investigations for more than a century. Of course we have some treatments, for example the wonderful hip replacement operations, but these help only to a minority of arthritis sufferers. For the majority, the medications we use to ease the suffering – steroids and non-steroidal anti-inflammatory drugs – carry a risk of unwanted side-effects that limit their use.

Any treatment that might help treat arthritis sufferers, particularly if it carries no risk of such side-effects, is very welcome news. But, as with many conventionally incurable diseases, false claims are often made. So the question is, will John Rowland's natural remedy really help arthritis sufferers?

I am sure that the reader's response, like my own, will be an initial scepticism. After years of affliction and doubt, who could blame arthritis sufferers if they despaired of ever finding the sort of relief offered in this book.

Yet in recent years there have been two developments in medical research which tend to support the thesis of this book. The first of these is the confirmation in several major trials that cod liver oil really does help sufferers from arthritis. Pure cod liver oil, a natural product, is now medically proved to relieve the joint pain and stiffness of rheumatoid arthritis. This interests me since, as co-author of *The Eskimo Diet*, I have long been convinced of the value of cod liver oil, both for alleviating the suffering of arthritis and in the prevention of heart attacks. The second development is the growing awareness within the medical establishment that diet can play an important part in relieving the inflammation of arthritis.

How interesting it is, therefore, that the two main principles of John Rowland's treatment – a treatment he has been using for thirty years, since long before the medical studies – correspond so closely to the latest results in orthodox medical research.

I wanted to know more about this and so I went to visit John Rowland to enquire in some detail into his clinical evidence and practical experiences with arthritis sufferers. I met a wonderfully unassuming man, calm, thoughtful and as organised in his approach as any medical colleague. I found a man who, only recently recovering from a life-threatening illness himself, was still determined to get back to work and to help others. I discovered that, through his very busy clinics in Blackpool and Marble Arch in London, he has given very real help to thousands of sufferers, including many well-known media and stage personalities. Indeed, I soon came to realise that this very kind and caring professional is one of the leading consultant herbalists in Europe, if not in the world.

But perhaps the most convincing recommendation for me – and also the best incentive for people with arthritis, particularly rheumatoid arthritis or rheumatism, to try John Rowland's course of treatment for themselves – is the huge number of letters of thanks he has received from sufferers he has helped all over the world.

CHAPTER ONE

My guiding philosophy

People who visit herbalists tend to have chronic conditions which have failed to respond to conventional medicine as prescribed by their doctor, and it is often in desperation that they turn to someone like me. They are sometimes so disillusioned that they have very little confidence left in their ability to cope with life, so the first thing I have to do is restore their confidence, both in themselves and in the possibility that herbal treatment might help them.

In the initial interview, I reassure prospective clients that herbal medicine is based on knowledge accumulated over thousands of years. At the same time, I have also to point out the limitations of herbalism. If I were involved in a car crash and required surgery of some kind then I would go to a surgeon for treatment; if I had any condition that would best be treated by the use of antibiotics then I would, and do, consult my local general practitioner. If, however, a condition is one of degeneration, like that of arthritis or psoriasis, then it is almost always worthwhile trying an holistic approach – herbal medicine integrated into a total health programme similar to the one explained in this book.

It may also be useful for the sufferer to continue taking some drugs prescribed by a doctor, as in an holistic approach it is not the means, but the end, which counts, and that end is eventual restored good health. The Chinese attitude to medicine is that the patient can receive either herbal or orthodox medicine or, if appropriate, both. Nobody gets upset because of professional pride; each profession is respected for the contribution it is making to the individual's total health programme.

Certainly the information in this book can be used in a number of ways. The holistic self-care programme described is designed specifically for the treatment of arthritis and can be followed at home, preferably in consultation with a family doctor. As an integral part of the treatment plan, detailed advice is given on how to eat sensibly and this can be used as a basis for healthy living generally.

Herbal medicine today

The theory and principles that I put forward in this book are not new. Plant medicine was one of the major sciences in the cultures of ancient China and Egypt. Now, thousands of years later, I am presenting you with similar principles in an effort to create a situation in which the body can heal itself. Our advantage over the Ancients is that we have the accumulated knowledge, ancient and modern, Eastern and Western, on which to base our treatment programmes.

As recently as the beginning of this century, almost all the medicines prescribed by doctors had their origins in the plant kingdom, many being dispensed in the form of extracts, pills, or infusions, as we suggest in this book. Herbal medicine was trusted because it had evolved over thousands of years of trial and error.

This implies no criticism of orthodox western medicine: indeed you need only stand in the outpatients' department of any hospital for a few minutes to be convinced of the need for drugs and surgery! Yet there is a movement throughout the world in favour of a revival of plant medicine, a desire for mild, natural cures which can be used in conjunction with an holistic approach to self-care.

The public has slowly come to realise that the most important defence against illness is the human body itself, and that it is the body's own defences that we should be helping wherever possible. The search for mild, effective medicines which have minimal side effects, are non-habit forming and can be used in a self-care system, has caused a world-wide resurgence of interest in herbs, vitamins, minerals and alternative therapies, a movement now so powerful that throughout the world it is being referred to as the 'green wave'.

Herbal medicines are natural substances derived from plants. They are often used by the plant itself for purposes such as defence against attack by insects or being eaten by other members of the animal kingdom. These *secondary plant products,* as they are called, are substances manufactured by the plant for that particular purpose and are therefore outside the main biochemical pathways of proteins, fats and carbohydrates. The current orthodox approach is to isolate the secondary plant products and try and define their specific action on the body, thence creating a new drug which is a purely chemical substance. It was this thinking which isolated the analgesic component of willow bark and thence produced aspirin; similarly, the curare herb, used by South American Indians to poison the darts for their blowpipes, has given doctors tubocurarine, used to relax muscles during anaesthesia.

Where the herbalist differs from orthodox medicine is in the use of the whole herb, or whole herb extracts, in the belief that secondary plant products are better administered to the body in the balance put there by nature. Herbalists refer to this as its *synergistic* form, which we believe will give the body all the benefits of the whole range of substances to be found in each plant.

This method carries fewer side effects and retains most of the benefits, particularly when used in conjunction with an holistic treatment programme such as the one advocated in this book. The variety of substances contained in a herb counters the potentially harsh effect of a powerful individual chemical. For example, the plant *ephedra* is used to treat asthma: the chemical ephedrine, which is the ingredient active against asthma, has the side-effect of raising the blood pressure, but other constituents of the plant, included in herbal preparations, counter the effect of the ephedrine on the blood pressure.

It is reasonable to suppose that secondary plant products will make valuable contributions to medicine in the future. There can be as many as a hundred secondary substances in any one plant and, given that there are over 350,000 known species of plant in the world, and so far we have only a cursory knowledge of about 10,000 of them, there is plenty of scope for research.

To help in this field, the World Health Organisation has established an institute in Rome for further studies. Many universities and teaching hospitals around the world are helping them with research and herbalists are contributing information. This pool of knowledge must help to advance the cause of natural medicine greatly in the coming years.

CHAPTER TWO

About arthritis

Arthritis is the commonest cause of disability in the United Kingdom, as in most developed countries of the world. Although it can afflict anybody at any age, the chances of being affected increase with age; over the age of 65 years an astonishing 41 per cent are affected. Over eight million people consult their doctors every year about some form of arthritic pain. It is clearly a very important disease.

It is also a very ancient disease; in one form or another, it has affected human beings throughout history. Indeed it is one of the oldest traceable diseases known to mankind and chronic spinal arthritis has been identified in the skeletons of the ape men of 2 million years ago.

Because we now know more about the disease, and have much better diagnostic techniques, the number of diagnosed cases has risen over the last few decades.

It was in the second century AD that Galen first grouped the rheumatic diseases together and called them arthritis but it was left to an English doctor called Garrod in the 1860s to differentiate between the two main conditions – rheumatoid and osteo-arthritis.

In this chapter, we will look at what is meant by arthritis, in both its forms.

Firstly, let me make it clear that arthritis is not a contagious disease like influenza or measles. There is a theory that people may inherit a predisposition towards the disease from their parents and that this tendency may be exacerbated by, for instance, infection, stress, fatigue, poor life style, toxic conditions, diet, draughts, work conditions, injury. Any bacterial disease, even when cured, may predispose to arthritis in later life, as can any of the other nine factors mentioned. The order in which these factors are listed is not significant; too few studies have been carried out to determine their relative importance. However, as with any total health programme, you should consider all these factors in relation to your own circumstances to see whether you can improve your lifestyle, for example by changing your diet or by reducing the amount of stress in your life, and thus make your chances of a successful cure that much better.

Forms of arthritis

Arthritis exists in many forms which are known by various names.

RHEUMATOID ARTHRITIS

This is a very important and common form of arthritis, characterised by a chronic inflammatory disease which affects various organs of the body, most obviously the joints. Two million people in the United Kingdom suffer from this in varying degree, an additional tragedy being the fact that 15,000 of these are children. Its onset varies from person to person, as does its immediate effects and the severity of its long-term effects. Joints that are affected may be swollen and painful with marked limitation of movement. After some years of damaging inflammation, the joints can become deformed, which makes the condition even more difficult.

Rheumatoid arthritis is undoubtedly one of the most unpleasant of all illnesses. Sufferers rarely have a day without pain. Very often many joints are affected, including most of the small joints of the fingers, the wrists, elbows, shoulders, hips, knees and ankles. The inflammation also extends beyond the joints to cause rheumatic pains in muscles and, in people severely affected, the painful and dangerous inflammation can extend throughout the body to include the eyes, the pleural membranes covering the lungs and even the membrane covering the heart.

Anybody who does not suffer from arthritis can hardly imagine what it is like to spend your day struggling with the simplest of tasks, such as turning a tap, opening a package or a can, doing the shopping or the housework – even tying your shoe laces. Sufferers may need special appliances to help them turn taps or even open doors. The joys of gardening may become impossible, though here again special adaptations can be very helpful. Anything that can be done to ease the pain, to lessen the stiffness, to allow the sufferer to return to work or to the fulfilment of their hopes and life is surely worthwhile.

UNDERSTANDING THE CAUSES

To understand the physiology of rheumatoid arthritis, one must first understand a little anatomy and then the chemical process of inflammation and degeneration which occurs when the body's immune system is either not coping or malfunctioning.

THE JOINTS

A joint is the flexible junction where two bones meet. The function of the joint is to allow a smooth and gliding movement of a limb. This is achieved by the encapsulation of two bone ends in a membrane called the *synovium*. In effect, the ends of the bones are encased in a sealed envelope which is filled with a lubricating fluid, called *synovial fluid*. Also present within this capsule are cushions between the bone ends to stop them grinding together. These cushions are made of a rubbery type of shock absorber called *cartilage*.

In an arthritic joint, the wearing out and degeneration of the bone ends is called *osteoarthritis*, while inflammation and destruction of the synovial membranes, with resultant eating away of the shock-absorbing cartilage is called *rheumatoid arthritis*.

THE AUTO-IMMUNE SYSTEM

The human body has a very complex system of defence against

infection and disease known as the immune system. It is organised and served by various organs and cells of the blood.

Normally if an invading bacterium, such as salmonella, or a virus, say the 'flu virus, enters the body, it is detected by the first line of defence: a type of white blood cell which may be a macrophage or a special type of lymphocyte.

The white cell's role is to distinguish anything it encounters in the blood or tissue as belonging to `self' or `non-self'. If it encounters `self', nothing occurs but when a foreign body or `non-self' item (`non-self' antigen) is found, the body's immune system is triggered and a sequence of events is set in motion.

Initially, the lymphocytes that have encountered and recognised this non-self antigen are stimulated and start to produce a series of chemicals, lymphokines, which have several major effects. Initially, these lymphokines work with the macrophages, whose job it is to eat and digest non-self antigens by a process known as phagocytosis: this effectively negates any harmful properties of the non-self antigen.

The lymphocyte's lymphokines also have the job of stimulating other cells into producing more chemicals: for example, the mast cells will release histamine. This release of further chemicals causes a localised constriction of blood vessels around the site of infection, producing swelling and the accumulation of blood and body fluids – thus an increased concentration of defending cells is created. This often causes an immobilisation of the area which is perceived by the senses as swelling, inflammation and stiffness.

The stimulated lymphocyte now undergoes a metamorphosis, changing into a much enlarged and aggressive cell known as a plasma cell whose function is to manufacture specific chemicals against the non-self antigens. These specific chemicals, known as antibodies, attack only this one particular non-self antigen: the antibody binds to the non-self antigen along with another blood chemical, called complement, and together they start destroying it. They also act as a beacon, signalling to the macrophages to eat and destroy it. In this the non-self antigen is neutralised and finally destroyed by these macrophages acting as vacuum cleaners and removing them from the body.

THE AUTO-IMMUNE SYSTEM AND THE JOINTS

In the person suffering from rheumatoid arthritis, an error has occurred in the first line of defence against the non-self antigens. For reasons we don't yet understand, the first line of defence in some persons has become confused and the normally helpful lymphocytes found within the synovial fluid perceive the bone ends or the synovial membranes as non-self antigens. Thus the body's defence system is put into action against these joint components which have been falsely identified as non-self antigens.

The lymphocytes produce their lymphokines which stimulate histamine release from the mast cells, thus causing swelling of the joints.

The lymphocytes metamorphose into plasma cells and produce antibodies against the bone or synovial membranes. The attracted macrophages start to eat and digest the bones or synovial membranes, causing inflammation and degradation of tissue. This is the explanation for what is happening inside the joint affected by rheumatoid arthritis. What you, the sufferer, notice is that the inflamed joint becomes swollen, stiff and painful to move, and eventually immobile. In severe cases, degeneration of the joint occurs, which wears out the joint surface in a very similar way to osteo-arthritis.

This attack on the bone or synovial membranes causes the classic symptoms of arthritis, but because the human body contains systems for repair of damaged tissue, it starts trying to repair the very tissue the immune system is destroying. It is important to understand this because it is this very process of self-repair that will be assisted by holistic healing. Thus an equilibrium between destruction and repair is struck. This equilibrium may be tilted in either direction by environmental factors or by the general state of health of the individual. Clearly, what we must aim for in treating arthritis is to tilt the equilibrium towards repair.

The mistaken release of the lymphokines and agents of defence against the membranes and bone unfortunately may not be localised to a specific joint: it may spread throughout the body in varying degrees as the agents of defence leak from the joint into the bloodstream and find new joints and membranes. In this way, a person with an arthritic knee may suffer with a stiff neck or sore chest. This is known as the systemic effect of arthritis and is the reason why the pain appears to move around the body from muscle to muscle and joint to joint.

EVEN AFTER SURGERY:

Where the joint has degenerated beyond the point at which one can reasonably expect the body's own repair mechanisms to work, surgery may be considered. Many people with very damaged hips or knees have found the surgical replacement of these damaged joints a wonderful blessing, relieving the pain of years and enabling them to get back into a more normal life. But even in these difficult circumstances, my natural remedy will continue to help you. The holistic approach is a total health programme which will assist in the recovery period and subsequently in slowing down any further degeneration of the bone.

ANTI-ARTHRITIS DRUGS

Certain forms of arthritis, such as gout, respond dramatically to modern drugs, but the common forms of arthritis, such as osteo and rheumatoid, are more difficult to treat in this way. Orthodox medicine does not claim to have found a cure for these forms, though drugs do often afford sufferers a good measure of relief from pain and other symptoms. Modern pharmaceutical science offers several types of such drugs which are taken by millions of arthritis sufferers throughout the world. Huge sums of money are spent every year on these drugs, commonly steroids and non-steroidal drugs aimed at reducing inflammation, which have been given the acronyn 'NSAIDS' (non-steroidal anti-inflammatory drugs). The medical profession does not regard these drugs as 'cures'. The difficulty with both these types of drugs is that they carry a risk of side-effects. For example steroids, if taken long term, can induce diabetes, thinning of the skin and suppression of the body's own glands, while the non-steroidals sometimes irritate the stomach, causing ulcers and other unpleasant complications.

I do not imply any general criticism of doctors or the pharmaceutical industry: they are doing their best to treat a serious and common illness. But even they will be the first to admit that the drugs commonly used for arthritis are far from perfect and they are continuing to search for better and less toxic treatments. In such circumstances, a holistic plan of treatment, without side-effects, has much to offer and it is hardly surprising that more and more people are turning to alternative medicine for treatment.

In a later chapter, we will discuss this holistic approach and how it may remedy the confused body response. Essentially, we look at the body as a whole and use every means in our power to restore a healthy equilibrium in all the body's functions. In particular we shall examine how combining the regular use of cod liver oil and herbs containing natural anti-histamines and anti-inflammatory and adrenal agents will help reduce pain and swelling while preserving the normal immune response to foreign invaders.

OSTEOARTHRITIS

This is the commonest form of arthritis and is really a wear-and-tear condition brought about by excessive use of one or more parts of the body, e.g. the finger joints or the weight-bearing joints such as the knees, hips and spine. The condition is slow to progress and very painful when the joint is used. Often the first signs are structural changes in the cartilage which loses its smoothness, with the consequence that the joint becomes stiff and sometimes immobile.

Unlike rheumatoid arthritis, osteoarthritis tends to affect only a small number of joints, usually the hip, the knee, the end joints of the fingers or the neck or lower back portions of the spine. It is mainly a condition of middle age and is more prevalent in women than men but it can occur at any age, particularly in sportsmen and women or people who have suffered some trauma, such as a car accident. Weight is best kept to a minimum for obvious reasons; the less weight the joints have to carry the better.

There are many practitioners who think this condition should be called osteoarthrosis because it is a wear-and-tear condition involving hardening of the joint as opposed to inflammation (`itis' denotes inflammation) which is rarely present.

Like rheumatoid arthritis, I have directed my natural treatment programme to helping people who suffer from this common and distressing condition.

Other forms of arthritis

BURSITIS

This is often called 'tennis elbow' or 'housemaid's knee' and is probably one of the earliest signs of a tendency to arthritis. It is caused by an inflammation of the bursa, a small sac which contains fluid and is usually situated between a tendon and the bone over which the tendon rides. This often occurs at the elbow and knee joints, hence the nicknames.

REITER'S SYNDROME

This is linked with arthritis and is a combination of conjunctivitis, or inflammation of the delicate membrane lining the eyelids, and urethritis, or inflammation of the tube draining the bladder. It usually affects young males for an indeterminate period ranging from weeks to months. It is a very painful condition.

FIBROSITIS

This is inflammation and soreness of the soft tissue of the body, as opposed to the joints specifically. It is often referred to as rheumatism, a term which covers a whole range of localised conditions brought about by some trauma, such as injury, or by pursuing a sport where there is a prolonged strain put on muscular tissue. It may also be referred to as backache or lumbago. It responds well to the sort of treatment discussed in this book; indeed it generally responds so quickly that it is rarely necessary to complete a full course of treatment. Adopting a healthy life style is a good basis to live by as, with any of the conditions that go by the name of rheumatism or fibrositis, there is always a predisposition towards arthritis.

IN SUMMARY

These are the conditions I treat with my natural remedy. Let us now take a look at the plan of treatment before hearing the experiences of many people whose lives have been helped by putting it into practice.

CHAPTER THREE

Explaining the programme of treatment

In essence, I shall be recommending a combination of two complementary treatments: a regular and effective dose of cod liver oil together with my special diet, which includes a course of treatment with herbs that have been tried and tested with hundreds of arthritis sufferers throughout my thirty years of experience as a consultant herbalist. I shall also outline some supplementary methods which will help give relief from pain and stiffness while you are waiting for the main programme to take effect.

Before getting down to the details of treatment, however, I would like to take this opportunity of explaining what holistic treatment is all about.

The general concept

In a nutshell, the general concept of holistic treatment is to create a condition, by means of diet, fasting, hydrotherapy, vitamin and mineral therapy, herbal medicine and usage of any other therapy that can assist the body's own healing process. As Hippocrates recognised all those years ago, 'the body is the prime physician'.

This is a successful way of controlling arthritis provided you have the necessary life force and determination to follow the programme through. It is based on an accumulation of clinical observations and handed-down knowledge from my predecessors at the naturopathic private clinic where I have worked with sufferers like yourself for thirty years.

The concept of the programme is simple: you first detoxify the body by eliminating from your diet as many as possible of the foods that may be causing your toxic condition. You use the unique properties of cod liver oil to reduce the inflammation in the joints caused by this toxic process while, at the same time, you use my diet and herbal treatment to clear away the toxins that have already accumulated in your body. You fast every seventh day and have special baths twice a week in between the fast days, in addition to your normal baths. After the special baths, you use a blend of oils to massage into the spine and affected areas.

To ensure that you are following the programme properly, I insist on a stipulated breakfast and lunch, but the evening meal is left very much to your own discretion. You are, however, given a guide to what you may or may not eat at this meal. This is my personally formulated 'Remedy Food Guide' and you will find it in a later chapter. Having sorted out the diet and the regular anti-inflammation doses of cod liver oil, so that the body is not only detoxifying itself but also regenerating, we help it along by the use of health foods, vitamins and minerals and herbal medicine. These are listed fully in Chapters nine and ten of this book.

Once we have set about the detoxification and supplementation programmes, we can then consider the various therapies which are available, to see which ones are likely to make an additional contribution to your self-care system. It may be allopathic drugs from your doctor, exercise, acupuncture, osteopathy, physiotherapy, your chiropractor or some form of electrical treatment. It does not matter which one or ones you choose, providing that each is making a positive contribution to the improvement of your condition. If you would like a simple analogy, think of each therapy in your self-care system as a tool in your anti-arthritis toolbox: use each tool as it is relevant to your immediate need.

It should be emphasised that undertaking your self-care treatment does not mean that you are no longer your general practitioner's patient. All it means is that you are assuming more responsibility for your own good health. It is my desire to work in tandem with your doctor to help you. I have little doubt that he or she would be interested in your progress and willing to help you along the way with counselling and whatever contribution he or she wishes to add to the natural remedy.

Perhaps this would be a good opportunity to explain what a herbalist means by detoxification.

Detoxification

One of the first concepts you must understand when beginning a self-care system of treatment is the principle of elimination and what is meant by the detoxification process which is so basic to the success of the programme. Fundamental to this is the fact that the body has four means of elimination: by faeces via the large intestine; by passing urine via the kidneys; by perspiration via the skin; and by exhalation via the lungs.

Herbalists believe that when the body's four means of elimination are not working properly, toxaemia results and this is the basis of most degenerative diseases. Simple forms of toxaemia are coped with by evacuation (by diarrhoea or vomiting), or by biliousness, when the liver returns toxins to the intestine via the bile duct. A more insidious form of toxaemia is when the liver is unable to cope with the poison and allows it to enter the bloodstream. The kidneys will be brought into play to filter the poison but if they are overworked they will have to call on the lungs to help out. We are all familiar with the person who has been drinking heavily and whose breath still reeks of alcohol. This occurs when the kidneys cannot cope and the lungs are brought into play.

When neither the kidneys nor the lungs are able to deal with the problem, then the skin and pores are called on to help eliminate and, in bad cases of drunkenness, to use the same example, body odour as well as breath odour can all too easily be detected. At this point, the body is just about coping in eliminating the excesses. To achieve this it must call upon the endocrine glands to release some of their hormones in order to reinforce the elimination process. If the body has to do this on a regular basis then an endocrine imbalance is often the outcome. In effect, the constant strain put upon the body in having to eliminate toxins results in the body becoming 'run down'.

This is the basis for most degenerative disease, because when the body's defences are down the virus or toxin can gain a hold. Sometimes nutrients are not available to the organs of the body so that more cells die than are created and so we get ageing or degeneration of that organ.

The first conditions to make themselves known are the minor ailments, the odd ache or pain and that feeling of being one degree under and not on peak form. After a period of time these minor ailments manifest themselves as various forms of arthritis, hypertension, various skin conditions such as psoriasis and eczema and various internal inflammations, such as bronchitis and colitis.

So what causes toxaemia? It depends on the particular susceptibility of the individual, but it could be alcohol, sugar, artificial food colourings, preservatives, drugs or one of many others. Apart from these, there are over 2,000 chemicals and additives that we may come into contact with in our daily lives without our knowledge – contained in such things as polishes, paints and glues, detergents, inks and so on. Stress can be another cause of toxaemia, often the last straw for the body's defences. One person will be more at risk than another from a particular toxin, and it is for this reason that an individual self-care system makes such good sense in the treatment of degenerative diseases.

What then is the best way to help the body use its own natural detoxifying methods? How can we best aid the processes of elimination?

The first thing to do, to ease the process of excretion, is to ensure that there is plenty of dietary fibre in our meals. Diets with a high fibre content have received a lot of publicity recently (though it should be said that nature-cure enthusiasts were until recently lone voices advocating this form of treatment) and it is easy to find out which foods are good in this respect. Wholewheat bread, whole grains and legumes, and plenty of fruit and vegetables are the prime factors. My Food Guide ensures that the intake of dietary fibre is adequate. The importance of fibre in the diet is that it acts rather like blotting paper when passing through the alimentary canal, taking up a lot of the debris and waste products. There is also the added benefit that it normalises the peristaltic action of the alimentary canal so that constipation is avoided.

After ensuring that we have sufficient dietary fibre, then we must look at our fluid intake to ensure that the kidneys are not being overworked or underworked. Remember that the kidneys are the blood's filters and the second of our four means of elimination. It is vital that we achieve the right quantity and quality of fluids in our treatment programme. I recommend lemon juice and water, or cider vinegar and water, to start the day, also the grape juice and water 24-hour fast every seventh day. Remember that water is nature's solvent and so, in the main, drinks based on water should be taken: these could be herbal teas such as chamomile, peppermint, rosehip or nettle – there are many to experiment with, such as parsley piert or dandelion which also makes a delicious coffee. I make this point about water-based drinks because I often find patients drinking juice only when on the programme and, though juices are permitted, they should not be taken in excess.

The next means of elimination is through the skin and its function of perspiration. It takes only a moment's thought to realise that the skin is the largest organ of the body. It has many physiological functions, but the one that we are most concerned with here is the ability to perspire and in so doing reduce the body's toxic build-up. This natural ability should be encouraged to the utmost and we achieve this in the programme by the use of hydrotherapy – the special baths.

These special baths should be taken at least twice a week. The sea salt which they contain combines many natural elements and has beneficial properties, not least of which are those of healing and antisepsis. The French are great supporters of thalassotherapy (the treatment of disease by sea bathing and sea air) and they have shown how many people who are suffering from various diseases can be helped by effective use of the sea's natural powers. We are not all in a position to get to a warm coast at a moment's notice, but we can add sea salt to our bath water and bring some of the sea's beneficial powers to our homes.

I shall give more details about the special baths in a subsequent chapter, but the general principle is that they should stimulate free perspiration. It is advisable to take your bath late, just prior to going to bed, when, after applying the oils to the spine and affected areas, you should wrap yourself in a bath robe to both aid and absorb the perspiration. The next day you will be pleasantly surprised at the invigorating effect of the bath and be ready to tackle your condition again.

The fourth method by which the body may eliminate toxins is by exhalation. We are all familiar with the person suffering from halitosis due to a gastric complication. The breath odour is caused by the body using the lungs as one way of detoxifying itself. It is with this in mind that the deep breathing exercises are recommended, aerobics if you are agile enough (but only under supervision), plenty of walking, which is my favourite, and swimming if your condition allows.

You will now have a basic idea of how detoxification works and will have begun to understand the importance of aiding this process when on a total health programme. Not only do we gain the benefit of a better oxygen supply to the bloodstream, and thereby the cells, but we also rid the body of the toxic build-up of salts and calcium which is necessary before we can begin to make progress on the healing programme.

Remember that a holistic programme is based on three premises. The first is to provide the body with all the nutrients that it could possibly need to put itself into good health. The second is to detoxify, removing all the poisons and accumulated debris from the system. The third is to improve the circulation so that the above two processes can work fully, with the cells receiving the nutrients and the waste products being carried from the cells and eliminated.

To achieve this threefold aim, we make full use of herbal medicine, regular cod liver oil treatment and vitamin and mineral supplements, hydrotherapy, exercise, and any other useful therapies available, in an effort to create a condition in which the natural healing processes of your body can work to your best advantage.

CHAPTER FOUR

The importance of cod liver oil

Our ease of access to our general practitioner is a relatively modern thing – indeed the notion of freely available healthcare only arrived in the United Kingdom in 1948 with the National Health Service. For hundreds and even thousands of years, most people were left to their own devices when it came to managing their health. For the most part the responsibility for health care fell to women. The mother, or the grandmother, in the family treated their kin.

Over this long history, a knowledge of treatments was acquired and was passed down from generation to generation by word of mouth. This is how both herbalism and orthodox medicine were born. Despite the intervention of great minds, such as Hippocrates and Galen in classical times, the burden of care continued to be the responsibility of the women in the family. Women accepted this responsibility as part of their role in providing the best from life for their children, their husbands and older or infirm members of the family or, more widely, their village or social group. As you might imagine, through many centuries of practice in this way, certain remedies emerged that were of real practical benefit, proven throughout many lifetimes of care. One of these remedies was and still is cod liver oil.

It seems likely that the health benefits of cod liver oil were first discovered by the wives of fishermen, whose arduous life and exposure to the elements made rheumatic complaints highly likely. A man afflicted by severe rheumatism could not go out to work. It would not take the wife of an afflicted fisherman long to realise that oily fish or the oil derived from the livers of white fish, such as cod, had a dramatic effect in relieving these rheumatic complaints. From the fishing communities, this knowledge filtered out into the general awareness, where it was taken up by the caring professionals, including herbalists and doctors.

The Romans are said to have used fish oil for a number of health-giving purposes, including the cure for hangovers. For many centuries, an awareness of the health-giving properties of cod liver oil preceded any scientific or medical understanding of how the oil worked. For example, when the British government discovered that more than half the young men recruited at the time of the Boer War were unfit for active service because of rickets, their medical advisers, knowing that regular cod liver oil would prevent rickets, put forward the idea that it should be made freely available to all children. Many will remember that regular morning spoonful from mother or grandmother, often made more palatable by being mixed with malt, which virtually abolished this disabling and disfiguring disease in the British population. It wasn't until many years later that vitamin D was discovered and it was then understood that cod liver oil was one of the best natural sources of this vitamin. Folklore and so-called "old wive's tales" had long preceded medical understanding.

Returning to arthritis, an interesting development began in the late eighteenth century when a Manchester doctor, called Samuel Kay, noticed the widespread faith in cod liver oil amongst ordinary people, particularly for rheumatism. Dr Kay went on to investigate the benefits of cod liver oil and subsequently used it to treat arthritis and rheumatism in very large numbers of patients.

In the 1930s an American army doctor, Ralph Pemberton, rediscovered the beneficial role of cod liver oil, which he used to help thousands of army personnel suffering from arthritis. He was before his time in establishing that cod liver oil worked best for arthritis and rheumatism when combined with a special diet.

An interesting chapter in the cod liver oil story took place when an eccentric but brilliant Oxford don, called Hugh Sinclair, visited the Inuit of Alaska in the 1940s. Sinclair had travelled from Britain to Canada for a different purpose entirely but while he was there he attempted to answer a question that had long puzzled him. The Inuit (or Eskimos) did not appear to suffer from heart attacks. At this time heart attacks were the new epidemic of the western world and Sinclair was convinced that diet was an important factor in the cause. Using a dog-sled, he visited the Inuit and confirmed they did not suffer from heart attacks. To his surprise, he also discovered that they did not suffer from arthritis, not even osteoarthritis, which we think of as associated with the wear and tear of ageing.

Over subsequent years, Sinclair performed experiments on himself which confirmed his belief that the healing properties in the Inuit diet was fish oil. His life and work pioneered the huge expansion of scientific studies of fish oil in universities, hospitals and other leading scientific institutions throughout the world.

Following Sinclair, more than a thousand scientific trials of fish oils in various illnesses have been performed. The results of such trials in arthritis have confirmed the long held belief of ordinary people that cod liver oil really does have unusual and highly beneficial properties for arthritis sufferers. Today some twenty-eight per cent of British people with arthritis use fish oil preparations, and pure cod liver oil is the leading medicine available without prescription for joint pain and stiffness. What new evidence for the treatment of arthritis has emerged from all of this scientific inquiry? And why and how does it work?

One of the first scientific studies looking at this was performed by two scientists called Brusch and Johnson in 1959. In this study, more than 90 per cent of arthritis patients given cod liver oil experienced a reduction of their pain and stiffness – and, what was just as interesting, their blood tests also showed significant improvement. This suggested that the cod liver oil was having a beneficial effect on the underlying mechanisms within the human body that led to arthritis. Another study, performed in 1986 and reported in the *Lancet*, concluded that some patients were so helped by eating oily fish that they were able to manage without drugs to treat their arthritis for up to four years. To understand why cod liver oil should have such properties, we need to look into the chemical changes that take place in our body when a joint becomes inflamed.

Most of us are aware that we should eat less saturated fat (the fat found in meat and full fat dairy produce) and eat more polyunsaturated fat (the oils found in vegetables and fish). What the new scientific research has shown is that these polyunsaturated oils in fish (special omega-3 fatty acids called EPA and DHA) are subtly different from the oils found in vegetables or any other dietary source. They are capable of switching off the chemical mechanisms within our bodies which lead to the formation of irritable chemicals, the very chemicals which give rise to inflammation in joints. Not only can they do this, they can also help to form quite a different form of chemical, which has the opposite effect of lessening inflammation. This may explain why cod liver oil reduces pain and inflammation in joints affected by arthritis – and particularly the stiffness that makes movement so very difficult first thing in the morning.

There is, of course, a salutary lesson here. For a long time science had refused to believe the experience of ordinary people. Scientists found it hard to come to terms with the fact that something as natural as cod liver oil could have dramatically effective healing properties. Perhaps this is why so many of the public now look more and more to complementary medicine for help. It would appear that alongside this pace of growth and change in modern life, has come an awareness for very many people, of the value of the ideas and experiences from that long and very practical past. Not least amongst these is the appreciation that our ancestors may have had a very sensitive understanding of the healing properties of substances derived from the natural world around them.

You will understand why I have made a point of including regular cod liver oil as an important ingredient in my natural healing programme.

The best way to take cod liver oil is in liquid form. If you find the taste difficult, I would suggest you mix it with twice the amount of cooled orange juice, lemon juice or milk and shake the mixture together for about 30 seconds. The dose I recommend is two teaspoons daily (one dessertspoon), or, if you have a chemist's measuring spoon, 10 ml. I have no objection to your taking it in the form of capsules if you prefer this.

Another useful tip is to first prepare your cup of tea or beverage of your choice, then drink your cod liver oil immediately before the first swallow of beverage. You soon get used to the taste and, within a week or two, will hardly need to mask it. You will also notice that I recommend that you take your cod liver oil last thing in the evening. This is to reduce that stiffness the following morning. But if you find it works best for you first thing in the morning, by all means take it then.

CHAPTER FIVE

The dietary concept

In my treatment programme there are several basic premises which I would like you to understand. The important role of cod liver oil has been outlined. Later in the book, I deal with individual foods, vitamins, minerals and herbs. Now I would like to outline the fundamental concept at the heart of the dietary part of your programme.

A good balance of amino acids, your body's basic building blocks, is essential; from this it will be able to synthesise its proteins. Secondly, a natural emulsifier is required to prevent the build-up of fats in the arteries. Thirdly, we should create as nearly as possible what I like to call a ninety-two element diet: a diet comprising all the elements of which the earth is composed and of which you and I are a part. Fourthly, every seventh day we should undertake a 24-hour fast.

Combining the above four principles with our modern knowledge about the effects of individual foodstuffs and elements on particular functions of the body, we can come up with a practical general guide as a basis for our diet programme. This guide reduces to an eight-point plan and, if you keep this in mind, you will not go far wrong in selecting suitable foods for yourself. Until you are completely familiar with the composition of the foods you eat, however, it is difficult to be sure that your diet is perfect in all respects and it is for this reason that, on the programme, the breakfast and lunch menus are stipulated, leaving only the evening meal to your own discretion. For the evening meal, you are asked only to follow the general guidelines and the eight-point plan which is as follows: higher potassium content; lower sodium content; low sugar content; low saturated fat content; high fibre content; high pantothenic acid (Vitamin B5) content; rich sources of nutrients; known peculiarities of certain foods.

Very briefly, the reasons for these criteria are as follows. Potassium is essential to the body and one of the main agents we are striving to increase in our health programme. The body's potassium level may be depleted, for example by the excessive use of sodium, sugar and caffeine, by using diuretics too often, or by the factor which so commonly underlies countless diseases – stress. People with arthritis, hypertension, leukaemia, heart disease, epilepsy and diabetes all have depleted potassium levels, often with correspondingly high levels of sodium. Most of the body's potassium is found in the cells, with a small amount in the body fluids and bloodstream. It has many roles to play, of which an important one is to help maintain a normal heart rhythm; others are the maintenance of muscle tone and the formation of extra bone, although its precise role in this is not fully understood.

At one time, there was a higher proportion of potassium than sodium in our diets and, indeed, the body adapted many of its own mechanisms to retain sodium: one of the functions of the kidneys is to ensure that the minerals are in the correct balance. However, there is such a high level of sodium in our present-day diets that our bodies are being overloaded with this mineral. In my diet, I help you to redress the balance in your food intake to a level that the body can cope with: I do not try to ban it altogether.

A cautionary word

This is a useful opportunity to emphasize the safety of the natural remedies I recommend. When I talk about increasing potassium and reducing sodium in your daily intake, I am, of course, talking about these elements as natural ingredients in food and not as medications. Potassium in drug form, for instance as potassium chloride tablets, is a different matter entirely. High doses of potassium as a medication should be treated as any other powerful drug and only dispensed under strict medical guidance.

People who suffer from impaired kidney or liver function need to be particularly careful with every ingredient in their diet, including potassium and sodium. Because of the kidney or liver impairment, they tend to accumulate excess sodium or potassium in their bodies so their diet should be individually worked out for them and closely monitored by a qualified dietician and kidney expert. I would not, therefore, recommend my diet to them. A simple rule of thumb will guide anybody who is at all uncertain. If you suffer from a medical complaint other than arthritis which involves special care with diet, you should discuss your intention of following my diet with your family doctor before starting it.

I aim to keep your sugar intake low so that the body is encouraged to obtain part of its energy from naturally balanced carbohydrates – the complex carbohydrates, rather than the simple carbohydrate found in refined sugar.

The refining of carbohydrate has created virtual powerpacks of concentrated energy – in fact many products are sold on just this point – but it is really only when undertaking strenuous exercise that this sort of energy source is required. Most of us should strive to obtain our energy requirements from a mixture of complex carbohydrates, fats and protein, all of which are interchangeable as far as the body is concerned as an energy source. We should avoid as far as possible the simple carbohydrates, such as dextrose, fructose and sucrose. Carbohydrate is, of course, essential to the human brain, nerve and lung tissue, and is supplied to these areas in the form of glucose. The main problem associated with a high intake of sugars is that the excess is converted to fats (triglycerides) and stored in the body in the adipose tissue as fat. On this programme, any excess fat is bound to create a problem and overweight can lead to all sorts of complications in your condition.

We strive on the programme to lower the overall intake of fats and to guide you towards the use of less saturated fats. Fats are composed of two basic types of fatty acids: saturated (hard) and unsaturated (soft, oil-like). Natural fats are a mixture of saturated and unsaturated fatty acids. The unsaturated fatty acids are so named because of the incomplete portions of the molecule (double bonds) and may have between one and six double bonds per molecule. Those with one double bond are known as mono-unsaturated and those with two or more double bonds are known as polyunsaturated; in this latter category are the essential fatty acids, such as linoleic and linolenic, which are required in small amounts for normal health but cannot be made in the body.

The greater the number of double bonds in the fat the more soft or oil-like is its consistency and, in order to incorporate these fats in foodstuffs and to give a product which has an acceptable appearance and consistency, it is necessary for manufacturers to hydrogenate or harden them. This involves saturating some or all of the double bonds to give a harder fat. The prime sources of these beneficial unsaturated fats is fish or cod liver oil and vegetable oils, with the major exceptions of palm and coconut oil, which are classed as saturated. The main source of mono-unsaturated fatty acids is oleic acid found in olive oil.

We should be trying also to reduce our intake of artificially-created, hydrogenated, fats. This is very convenient for the food-producer who can thus virtually dictate the shelf-life of his product, but the end product is by no means ideal for us and should be avoided as much as possible.

The reasons for a high fibre intake have been discussed in the chapter on detoxification, but I would like to add here that evidence is accumulating all the time to support the advisability of adopting a diet rich in fibre such as bran. Oat bran, for example, contains an agent called beta-glucan, which carries cholesterol to the colon, and serious medical conditions such as haemorrhoids, diverticulitis, varicose veins, colitis, cancer and atherosclerosis can all be attributed in some degree to a long-term lack of fibre in the diet.

Pantothenic acid (vitamin B5) is essential for the proper dispersal of fats, carbohydrates and proteins. It plays a major role in the creation of amino acids and steroid hormones and it is for this main reason that it is an important ingredient of our programme.

In our treatment programme, it is essential that we provide the body with the raw materials from which it may select its own requirements and, for this reason, it makes sense to include in our diets foods which are rich sources of nutrients. Kelp, for example, contains many minerals and we would do well to study which foods are good sources of some of the more obscure minerals, such as manganese.

In the Food Guide, I have taken into account clinical observations on patients suffering from arthritis and I have listened to the opinions of patients who have learned through trial and error which foods, food colourings and preservatives and methods of preparation are counter-productive. The Food Guide reflects a balance of evidence for and against certain substances. Remember, however, that the essence of the self-care programme is that it is individually tailored and you will have to observe very carefully the effects of all foods and food substances on your own condition.

As it is important that you should fully understand the reasons behind the diet programme, let us now look in more detail at the fundamentals of the regime; the inclusion of amino acids, an emulsifier, the 'ninety-two element diet' and the fast.

Amino acids are, as already mentioned, the body's basic building blocks and they are obtained from our intake of protein. There are twenty-two of them, ten of which are essential to life.

Unlike plants, which can manufacture their own proteins, we need to obtain proteins from food and it is essential that we have a regular intake of complete proteins from such things as lean meats, fish, eggs, fowl, milk, cheese, buttermilk, yoghurts, soya beans, nuts, beans, peas, yeast and grains. As the egg has a near-perfect balance of amino acids, other sources of protein are compared with it as a reference standard. Unfortunately, the kidneys may have difficulty in coping with the high albumin content of eggs, so you should not have more than three eggs a week. Also there is the point that your amino acid intake is best obtained from a variety of sources; this will enable your body to manufacture thousands of different proteins from the different amino acids broken down by the enzymes in the digestive process.

These amino acids are carried around the body by the bloodstream and are selected by the cells for use in the production of new body tissue and replacement of such important substances as antibodies, hormones, enzymes and blood cells. It is easy to see that a long-term shortage of protein creates a condition in which degenerative disease can easily set in. It should be mentioned in passing that a very high intake of protein over a long period can also be injurious to health; damage in the form of nephritis, or Bright's disease, can occur. Our need for protein varies very little whether we are at work or rest and any excess over and above that needed for replacing the body tissue, puts a strain on the kidneys. In the stipulated diet, and following the eight-point plan for the selection of food, you should run no risk of overconsumption of protein.

The second fundamental ingredient in our diet after amino acids is a natural emulsifier in the form of an element called lecithin. It is included as one of the regular ingredients of the breakfast in the treatment programme.

Most people will be aware of the danger of cholesterol deposits on the walls of the arteries. These deposits not only impede the flow of fresh, nutrient-rich blood to the cells but also become a danger to good health in themselves as the cause of heart disease. We must take steps in our diet not only to prevent the build-up of fat deposits, but also to clear away what is there at the present time.

Although cholesterol is always given a bad press, I should mention that it is constantly manufactured in the body by the liver in the right amounts to make vitamin D and the hormones and bile salts it requires. We get into difficulties because our diet is high in saturated fats from animal sources, dairy produce and processed foods containing hard or saturated fats and hydrogenated oils.

If the body finds no use for these globules of fat, they gather together in deposits called atheroma on the artery walls and become the initial cause of conditions like high blood pressure, hardened arteries, heart attacks and strokes. A very welcome added bonus from cod liver oil is its protective function against this hardening of the arteries.

What is also needed to break down these clusters is an emulsifier, a substance which acts as a sort of soap. Vegetable oils, such as sunflower and safflower, are bonded with lecithin, nature's strongest emulsifier, whose job it is to break down the globules of fat into small particles so that they are ready to be absorbed by the tissues when required. As well as supplementing the diet with lecithin in granule form, it is wise to restrict the intake of fat to the polyunsaturated kind. It is interesting to note, as a bonus, that lecithin contains two important vitamins of the B complex, choline and inositol, essential to the brain, nerves, heart, lungs and in the production of certain hormones. It is also gaining a reputation as an agent that can prevent senile dementia.

The third premise on which our treatment programme is founded is that we should approach as nearly as possible a `ninety-two element diet'. The elements referred to are trace elements, substances essential to plant or animal life but present in only very small amounts. There are at least ninety-two of them and they make up the basic composition of the earth and everything in it. In that the same concentrations of salts and trace elements that make up our blood and tissues were found in the earliest seas – the primaeval soups – we can indeed be called the children of the earth. The nitrogen in the atmosphere that is 'fixed' by conversion in the soil into nitrates to feed plants is the same nitrogen that is part of the connective tissue that binds our bones together, just as the calcium in our bones is the same as the calcium that forms the rocks of our hills and mountains.

If we organise ourselves properly, then we should never be

short of minerals as they are available in abundance. But here it is worth drawing attention to an obvious and balanced source of many nutrients. While we are still not sure what life is, we can at least see for ourselves the first act of growth of an embryo plant – the sprouting or germination of the seed. Although to sustain growth, it will need nutrients from water, soil and air, this initial surge of activity is supported entirely by the miniature chemical factory called the seed, in which all the natural elements are contained in the right proportions. As it is a source of balanced nutrients that we are trying to capture in our diet, it must make sense to include a high proportion of these basic forms of life; seeds, whole grains and legumes.

Fourthly, and finally as a general principle, a 24-hour fast is part of the treatment programme. The thinking behind this is that the body needs a period in which the elimination processes may be helped, and that the kidneys can have a chance to utilise the healing and diuretic properties of grape juice over that period. The Swiss have long regarded grape juice as a way of avoiding kidney stones, and the maintenance of healthy kidneys is one of our main aims on the programme.

The easiest way to achieve a 24-hour fast is to miss the evening meal of one day and the breakfast and midday meal of the next. The gap in eating is then spread over two days and no single day is spent without food.

CHAPTER SIX

The living proof

There will be stages in the programme which follows when it is difficult to believe that you are making any progress, and it is for this reason that I now include some comments from my patients which demonstrate typical feelings at various stages of the treatment and, happily, typical relief at the eventual cure. The letters are representative of the many hundreds I have received from people who have attended my clinic and have derived benefit from the system of medicine I have evolved over the years into one of total health and self-care, relevant, with variations, to the treatment of many ailments, including psoriasis and hypertension. To use a system of this nature requires effort, but the reward of good health it brings is priceless.

Virtually all the people who come to me have tried treatment by orthodox medicine and, although the treatment may have failed, it is in fact very helpful to have, in every case, a confirmed diagnosis. The type of treatment used prior to the consultation with me is also on record and it is very helpful for me to have a positive relationship with the patient's medical adviser, though unfortunately this does not always develop.

Some points you should note when reading the letters are the different times it takes to see results; the amount of tablets and liquid medicine taken; and the importance of good nutrition to the success of the programme. Details of stockists can be obtained from the Naturopathic Private Clinic (address in appendix).

At the Naturopathic Private Clinic, I have clients from as far afield as the USA, South Africa, Nigeria and Saudi Arabia, which is amazing when you consider that no advertising is undertaken, all recommendation being by word of mouth.

Following a discussion with one of my clients, Mrs H. decided that a natural treatment was also for her. She consulted her doctor, who had no objections and, indeed, co-operated by monitoring her progress on the programme. He gradually reduced her treatment for arthritis and hypertension as her condition improved.

> *I had suffered with arthritic knees for over twenty years, during which time my doctors gave me various tablets which helped ease the pain. Then unfortunately I developed colitis and could not take any [painkilling] pills as these aggravated this condition. I also started to suffer from high blood pressure and had to start taking tablets which my doctor said I would have to take for the rest of my life. The arthritis became much worse: going upstairs, walking up even slightly hilly streets, and kneeling became a bit of a nightmare, and I grew tired and depressed with the effort. I also got increasing pain in my shoulders, arms and top of my spine which kept me awake most nights. At this stage a friend of mine recommended Mr Rowland and he put me on a programme to which, I am thankful to say, I responded. This was two years ago and now I can get about and kneel much more readily. Though I do get twinges of pain, I haven't had a really bad day, with that terrible pain all arthritis sufferers know, for over six months. As an added bonus, the colitis is under control, and so is the high blood pressure. I haven't taken a tablet for high blood pressure for over twelve months: my doctor says that the treatment from Mr Rowland is keeping that under control.*

Mr V. M. has written a very descriptive letter which needs little further explanation, other than to re-emphasise the importance of sticking to the system as strictly as possible and reaping the rich rewards of good health by doing so.

> *It is almost six months since I visited the Naturopathic Clinic to consult Mr Rowland about osteoarthritis which had started to disable me seriously. My feet, legs and hips were*

painful, the pain extending down my legs and up to my left shoulder and arm. I was unable to sleep and had become almost immobile. The pain was such that I was unable to pick up a cup of tea with my left hand. For four months prior to my consultation with Mr Rowland I had received tablets from my doctor, but as my condition continued to deteriorate I discontinued the tablets. Mr Rowland prescribed dietary changes, fasting one day a week, herbal medicine, vitamin and mineral therapy and massaging with Rowlo Oil. After one month of treatment the pain was less intense so that I was able to sleep, and there was a noticeable improvement in my foot joints. After two months the range of movement in my left arm was considerably better and the pain in my left arm was not so severe. There is now no pain at all in the foot joints. The only areas of pain which remain are the knees, lower back, and hip joints. After three months I had the full range of movement back in my left arm and shoulder, with only slight pain on waking in the morning. I still have some pain in my back and hip joints but this is considerably less than when I started the treatment. After four months there was only slight pain in my back and hip, and shoulder areas. After almost six months improvement continues. I can walk at almost my old speed, and at sixty-two years of age can move faster than many half my age. The occasional pain I have is only slight.

If you have rheumatoid arthritis then read the following letter often as it will give you the heart to tackle the condition. Even by keeping to the programme which follows you will find it a battle to overcome the condition. I cannot offer a miracle, merely the means to fight which in itself often results in restored health.

Using my programme, Mrs D. was taking a large quantity of tablets and vitamins: this often comes as a surprise to people not previously acquainted with this sort of holistic treatment. There are many reasons for the large quantities of herbal tablets often required and one is that, because the fibres of the plant are left in the tablet, any one tablet contains very little of the active ingredient. Fibres are left in so that, as the tablet disintegrates in the stomach, a bulky area is created from which the body can extract its requirements. This system means that there will be few or no side effects from what may be a very potent herb: it is this principle on which most of my herbal tablets are formulated.

The other points to look for when reading Mrs D's letter are firstly, the length of time it took for the detoxification to work before any real progress was made, and secondly, how her vitality was at a low ebb for some considerable time. Gradually, however, the rewards started to come, vitality was restored and the healing process gathered momentum.

Mrs D.'s letter starts with a description of the years of pain she suffered from rheumatoid arthritis and the drug therapy with its misery of side-effects and addiction. At the point when her doctors wanted to use yet another drug to help wean her off steroids she turned, at the age of thirty-one, to herbal medicine. It was an uphill struggle, as she first had to overcome her dependence on Prednisolone. She continues:

> With the herbal method certain items were excluded from my diet: white flour, hard fats, white sugar, caffeine and salt. Tablets and medicine were prescribed, special baths were recommended, and I slowly reduced the dose of Prednisolone. After four months I ceased to take Prednisolone at all. I had to suffer all the pains of withdrawal, especially in my back, neck and shoulders, and stiffness in my joints was not confined to mornings, but occurred sometimes during the day as well, being very much in evidence by early evening. This stage lasted for over three months. I needed analgesics during this period and I was very weak, the slightest exertion leaving me shaky and breathless. My tablets were changed, the pain and stiffness ceased, and I felt much better. I was able to begin full-time work.
>
> The tablets and medicine were again changed after about six months but did not suit me, and after a while the treatment

was changed yet again. In another four months my health was slowly improving, my progress becoming steady. My strength increased and I was at a stage where I could sleep peacefully at night, with only a little stiffness in the mornings, this being wonderful when I think of the time when I had to be helped out of bed. I had greater freedom of movement – once I could not bend down, had difficulty rising from a sitting position and climbing stairs, and even experienced pain in my jaws when eating.

Now four years later my good condition is being maintained and the crippling disease is kept well in control. I am hopeful for the future once more. The people around me seem to have forgotten my illness, although they only knew me after my treatment had started to work: if only they could have seen me in earlier years they would realise that I am indeed living proof that herbal medicine really works.

There is a world of difference in the two types of treatment that I have received – the conventional way with drugs, that I have personally found useless in the long term; and the naturopathic way without harmful side effects and which rebuilds health and strength, revitalising the system.

The interesting point about the success of this next case is that it is the result of a joint effort between myself and the patient's doctor, because she is still on a drug that she finds useful and her doctor prescribes it for her in conjunction with my treatment. My only regret is that her doctor was not standing with me on the first day that she walked from her car leaving her wheelchair behind, a very emotional moment that had my staff crying with joy. The letter which follows is from the client's husband.

Five years ago my wife started to suffer with rheumatoid arthritis; she became very disabled, having to use a wheelchair, and she started to stoop. Her arms and legs were very bad. I did not believe in herbalism, but my wife begged me to take her, and so in the end I gave in. After eighteen months' treatment under

Mr Rowland my wife got back the use of her left arm and left leg,
and – owing to the skill of Mr Rowland – the arthritis is
contained in her left side only, and there is a big improvement in
that. Before the start of this treatment my wife could not do
anything with her arms, and could not walk a step. Now the
stoop is going and she can move her arms; the most amazing thing
to me is that she can now walk about 50 yards.

The most interesting aspect of the next letter is how *Dr Dong's*
Arthritic Cookbook was being followed with some success but was too
severe a regime to stick to for long. This may be the case for some
people with my programme and, if in your self-care treatment you
feel that you need some encouragement, go without delay to a
practitioner who has experience of this type of treatment.

Up to the time I consulted Mr Rowland I had been
prescribed pain-killing drugs which relieved the pain of arthritis
for only a limited time. I was completely unable to use my hands,
drive the car or walk without help. I then heard of Dr Dong's
Arthritic Cookbook and decided to give it a try: after three
months most of the pain had gone, along with the swelling, but I
didn't feel any better in myself, and I knew that the diet was one I
would never be able to keep to. It was at this point that I decided
to pay Mr Rowland a visit: I was very confused about the
properties of certain foods and medicines and needed the advice of
an experienced practitioner. I had been led to believe that calcium
was taboo, as was fruit, but I now know that grapes and
pineapple play a big part in helping arthritis, and that calcium
pantothenate (Vitamin B5) is essential as it produces necessary
hormones and converts carbohydrates into energy.

The salient point of the next letter is contained in just two
sentences but is a very important message:

After a few months on Mr Rowland's treatment I found it
hard to believe that my worsening symptoms were actually part of
the cure, and they would get worse before they got better.
However, they gradually abated and I have got better and better,

*so much so that I now no longer think about my ailments at all
and it is difficult to remember how bad they actually were, and
how much they got me down.*

I leave the last word to Mrs C., who has been attending my clinic for some years now. When she first came to the clinic her osteoarthritis was quite severe and she was hardly able to walk. Although her progress has been slow it has been steady and now, at the age of 71 years, Mrs C. is living a full and active life, her chief enjoyment being ballroom dancing. The holistic self-care system treats the whole person, restoring vitality and the quest for a new life – which can include ballroom dancing at 71!

*I had been under the doctor for six years suffering from
osteoarthritis. I could not walk very much and had a lot of pain.
A friend of mine was going to Mr Rowland and took me along:
within six weeks I was a little better, and within twelve months I
was dancing. I am still dancing at the age of seventy-one.*

CHAPTER SEVEN

The programme

I have developed this programme of treatment after experience with many hundreds of cases of arthritis of varying degrees of severity. I have found that six distinct stages of progress are involved and the preparations suitable for each stage are different. In the following pages, I outline in brief what you can hope to experience at the six stages. I then give the breakfast and lunch menus to be used throughout the programme; and then deal with the preparations to be used at the six stages of treatment. Further details of the herbal ingredients are given in the appendix.

The six stages of progress

1. A feeling that you are more lively and more able to cope with your condition, although the pain has not yet lessened.
2. You are sleeping better and the pain is starting to localise to two or three places.
3. This is a period of very little change and there may even be a slight worsening of the condition, though this will rarely be as bad as before the programme started. This stage may last for several months.
4. A more confident feeling and a slow realisation that you have more mobility.
5. The confidence grows and the pain has almost gone, but there may still be evidence of it in the local areas.
6. Your confidence is fully restored and you start to get bored with

the programme. You can gradually come off the strict guidelines without any ill effects and, because of your re-educated attitude, you will not make many dietary errors in future. I do however advise you to be prudent with your diet for life and to take a regular dessertspoon of cod liver oil as a preventive or control measure throughout your life.

The regular menu

On rising

1 tablespoon of lemon juice in a small glass of water. Bottled lemon juice is acceptable, though I prefer the freshly squeezed lemon if available.

Cod liver oil tip: If you prefer to take your cod liver oil in the morning, this would be a good opportunity to follow the cod liver oil with the lemon juice or even mix the two by shaking together for 30 seconds before swallowing.

Breakfast

1 tablespoon wheatgerm
1 tablespoon lecithin granules
1 tablespoon muesli or porridge
1 teaspoon molasses
1 teaspoon bran
1 teaspoon honey
Skimmed milk
Wholemeal toast with honey or molasses
Dandelion coffee or decaffeinated coffee

Lunch

Salad with plenty of grated root vegetables and sprouting seeds
Fresh fruit (not citrus, except lemon)
Herbal tea
Glass of wine if desired

Evening meal
A good starter is unsweetened pineapple juice.

The rest of the meal is left to your own discretion, but you must follow the general guidelines of the Food Guide, as given in Chapter nine.
It is acceptable to transpose the evening menu with the lunch menu.

Bathing and fasting
There are two particular aspects of the programme that need to be mentioned here.

Special baths
Twice weekly you should take a special bath, as discussed in Chapter three. Add to the bath water ½lb (250g) sea salt, ½ lb (250g) Epsom salts and ½oz (15g) powdered culinary ginger. Keep the temperature of the water as high as you can stand throughout the bath by topping up while you are soaking.
When you get out of the bath, lightly dry yourself and apply Rowlo Oil to the whole of the spine and affected areas (I will give you the formula for this oil on page 77). Then wrap yourself up well and retire to bed where, hopefully, you will perspire, so aiding the elimination process.

FASTING

You should fast for 24 hours every seventh day, drinking only grape juice and water.

The way to achieve this is to extend the natural fasting period of sleep and miss the evening meal on day one, and breakfast and lunch on day two. You will thus create a period of 24 hours without food, but no single day passed without eating.

You do not take any preparations during this 24 hour period, but you do have the ones that go with the meals before and after the fast.

Please note in particular that you should keep up the fast all the time you are on the programme, that is, throughout the six stages; you should not have a special bath during the fast period; you may, if you feel at all light-headed during the fast, have a few grapes as well as the grape juice and water.

Stage One

When you first start taking the preparations as outlined below you may suffer some digestive upset. As my old tutor used to say, 'It is like stirring up a still pond'. If this occurs, go on to the preparations gradually so that you are taking the full amount by the end of the second week. Take the preparations after food and, in the case of the morning and evening meals, take them with the drink made from the tisanes.

I hope that you will have discussed with your doctor your intention to undertake this programme of treatment and that he or she will co-operate by monitoring your progress for you. It is to be hoped that during this first stage of the programme you can try coming off any anti-inflammatory or pain-killing drugs your doctor may have been prescribing for you.

During this stage you should be getting into the habit of taking the special baths and undergoing a 24-hour fast every seven days. You will be living with these two aspects of the regime for some time, so some experimentation now with which days of the week best suit your lifestyle will pay dividends over the months.

You should stay on the first stage preparations for at least 30 days before moving on to Stage Two.

STAGE ONE PREPARATIONS

After breakfast
2 Multivitamin and Mineral Formula
I Vitamin C Plus 500 mg
Parsley Sprinkle
2 Kelp Tablets
Celery Compound Tisane Drink

After lunch
2 Pantothenic Acid 500 mg
2 Kelp Tablets

After evening meal
Parsley Sprinkle
1 Pantothenic Acid 500 mg
2 Kelp Tablets
Celery Compound Tisane Drink

On retiring
2 Meadowsweet and Willow Bark Compound

Your evening cod liver oil

I usually recommend that my patients take a dessertspoon of cod liver oil on retiring because I have found this helps avoid the morning pain and stiffness. As mentioned earlier, it is quite permissible to take it in the morning if you prefer to do so. If the taste is a problem for you, I have given some tips on how to mask this at the end of Chapter Four: The importance of cod liver oil.

Stage Two

At this stage you will see that an increased amount of Pantothenic Acid is stipulated. Also during this stage you will find that the pain will localise and it is on these local points that you should use the Rowlo Oil. You will find that the pain will be different at different times of the day and, if it becomes difficult to bear, you may take up to nine Meadowsweet and Willow Bark Compound tablets per day.

This stage will probably go on for 16 to 18 weeks, after which you may well find yourself at something of a standstill. This signifies the beginning of Stage Three, which is a very important one in the programme.

STAGE TWO PREPARATIONS

After breakfast
2 Multivitamin and Mineral Formula
1 Vitamin C Plus 500 mg
Parsley Sprinkle
2 Kelp Tablets
2 Pantothenic Acid 500 mg
Celery Compound Tisane Drink

After lunch
2 Kelp Tablets
2 Pantothenic Acid 500 mg

After evening meal
Parsley Sprinkle
2 Kelp Tablets
2 Pantothenic Acid 500 mg
Celery Compound Tisane Drink

On retiring
1 dessertspoon Cod Liver Oil

N.B. You may take up to nine Meadowsweet and Willow Bark Compound tablets per day if the condition is still painful.

Stage Three

In Stages One and Two you will have been feeling the benefits of the vitamin, mineral and herbal preparations as well as improved nutrition from following the food guide. Hopefully, you will have been able to stop any toxic medication. This is the point at which the liver will be leading the body to complete detoxification and there may well be withdrawal symptoms and a regression in your condition during this period.

Even if you were not on any prescribed drugs, your body has been asked to do without food substances such as caffeine, sugar and a high salt intake that it may have been used to all your life. These may be the agents that your body is now craving.

It is very important not to weaken in your resolve to attain good health and you should, if anything, become more rigorous in following the Food Guide.

During Stage three, which may go on for weeks or months, the preparations change considerably. African Devil's Claw and Jamaican Sarsaparilla are introduced for the first time, and the tisanes change to a formula based on dandelion. You may wish to refer to Chapter Ten for more information about these substances.

STAGE THREE PREPARATIONS

After breakfast
2 Multivitamin and Mineral Formula
1 Vitamin C Plus 500 mg
1 Pantothenic Acid 500 mg
Parsley Sprinkle
Dandelion Herbal Compound Tisane Drink

After lunch
1 Pantothenic Acid 500 mg
2 African Devil's Claw and Jamaican Sarsaparilla Compound Tablets

After evening meal
1 Pantothenic Acid 500 mg
2 African Devil's Claw and Jamaican Sarsaparilla Compound Tablets
2 Kelp Tablets
Dandelion Herbal Compound Tisane Drink

On retiring
1 dessertspoon Cod Liver Oil

N.B. Up to nine Meadowsweet and Willow Bark Compound Tablets per day may be taken for pain relief.

Stage Four

You will now have a more confident feeling and your mobility will increase. In particular, your arms may well feel lighter and have more movement.

Together with this greater mobility and increased confidence may come an unexpected pain, and this is the pain of freedom. Your blood circulation will have improved and you will have been through the major part of the detoxification process. There will, however, still be some residual toxic waste in the joints and this will cause pain as you begin to make use of your greater mobility. Do not let this pain concern you; your body will deal with this residual waste matter in good time as long as you persevere with the programme. In the meantime, you may find it helpful to take an additional special bath and to apply the Rowlo Oil more frequently.

STAGE FOUR PREPARATIONS

After breakfast
2 Multivitamin and Mineral Formula
1 Vitamin C Plus 500 mg
Parsley Sprinkle
Celery Compound Tisane Drink

After lunch
1 Vitamin E 200 i. u.
1 Pantothenic Acid 500 mg

After evening meal
1 Pantothenic Acid 500 mg
2 Kelp Tablets
Parsley Sprinkle
Celery Compound Tisane Drink

On retiring
1 dessertspoon Cod Liver Oil

N.B. Up to nine Meadowsweet and Willow Bark Tablets per day may be taken if there is still any pain.

Stage Five

Your confidence will grow markedly during this period as the pain abates and, though there may be some localised pain, your whole general health will be so much improved that you will feel well able to cope.

At this stage you should start to reduce your intake of preparations. I find that people generally find it most tiresome to remember the preparations after the midday meal, so it is probably best to discontinue these first.

STAGE FIVE PREPARATIONS

After breakfast
1 Multivitamin and Mineral Formula
1 Vitamin C Plus 500 mg
Parsley Sprinkle
Celery Compound Tisane Drink

After lunch
None

After evening meal
2 Pantothenic Acid 500 mg
2 Kelp Tablets
Parsley Sprinkle
Celery Compound Tisane Drink

On retiring
1 dessertspoon Cod Liver Oil

N.B. If any pain remains Meadowsweet and Willow Bark Tablets may be taken as required, up to a maximum of nine per day.

Stage Six

At this point you will have achieved a state of relatively good health. You will have become bored with the programme and you can start to come off it. The best way to do this is gradually to relax your lifestyle and not make as many errors as before. In part the programme is educational and, by this stage, you will have found out which of the foods and preparations are most suitable for you.

I recommend that you take the vitamins and minerals and the Celery Compound Tisane Drink at a maintenance level to supplement your diet, plus any of the other preparations that you feel did you the most good. The cod liver oil should be taken indefinitely, since it not only keeps down the inflammation but helps to prevent the arthritis coming back.

STAGE SIX PREPARATIONS

After breakfast
1 Multivitamin and Mineral Formula
1 Vitamin C Plus 500 mg
4 Kelp Tablets
Celery Compound Tisane Drink

After lunch
None

After evening meal
Any of the preparations that you used in the programme that you felt did you the most good.

On retiring
Celery Compound Tisane Drink
1 dessertspoon Cod Liver Oil

The quick "Rheumapainaway" programme

Many people with minor rheumatic complaints may not require the complete programme of treatment and for these I have formulated a much simpler programme, as follows:

Cod liver oil
1 dessertspoon at night (or morning if preferred). See advice on how to take it in Chapter Four.

Vitamins and herbal treatment
1 Nutra Tone for two months
1 Vita Vitality for the third month
9 Rheumapainaway capsules: 3 capsules three times daily, reducing to 3 capsules daily. These work by stimulating the natural resistance to pain of the body's endorphines
3 Calcium Pantothenic daily, taken as a 500 mg tablet three times daily.

Rheumapainaway oil
Rub into the joints twice a day.

CHAPTER EIGHT

Additional treatments that may help you

The holistic approach

To remind you of the general concept of holistic treatment, we are looking to create a condition whereby the body can heal itself. In addition to the very important subject of diet, we can select from the variety of therapies which are available to aid blood circulation and the efficient function of heart and lungs. Some therapies, such as acupuncture, osteopathy, or chiropractic may also directly alleviate pain and they should be used where they can be helpful to our programme. Before undertaking an holistic programme you should have a confirmed diagnosis of your condition from your doctor and his approval of the therapies you intend to use. You should review your self-care programme and take further medical advice if any sudden change occurs in your condition, particularly in the heart or lung function. In addition, you should not continue with any aspect of your programme which you approach with a negative attitude so that you doubt its worth.

In the main programme of treatment, I recommended the use of hydrotherapy, special baths and aromatherapy (the massage of oil into the skin). There are many other therapies that could help you and I shall devote a little time to explaining these. They include deep breathing, exercise, homeopathy, acupuncture, osteopathy, chiropractic, physiotherapy or some form of electrical treatment. In addition, you may wish to use some allopathic drugs from your doctor.

Let us take a look in turn at each of these possibilities, starting with the ones I recommend in the main programme.

HYDROTHERAPY

The idea behind the special baths is that they should stimulate free perspiration, thus aiding the process of elimination. In this arthritis programme, they are recommended twice weekly.

Have the bath water as hot as you can stand and add to it ½ lb (250g) sea salt, ½ lb (250g) Epsom salts and ½ oz (15g) powdered ginger (ordinary culinary ginger). Keep the temperature of the bath water high by topping it up while you are soaking. Stay in the bath for at least 20 minutes.

When you get out of the bath, lightly dry yourself and, with the help of an assistant if necessary, apply Rowlo Oil to the whole of the spine and the affected areas (see the section below on aromatherapy). Then wrap yourself in a bath robe and retire to bed where you should perspire freely, aiding the elimination process.

As already mentioned, the properties of sea salt are many and varied. It is included in the special bath principally for its healing and antiseptic properties. Ninety-eight per cent of known germs are unable to survive longer than 48 hours in sea water. The Epsom salts are included because of their healing and drawing properties when combined with sea salt, and the ginger has the property of toning the skin and stimulating perspiration, which is the aim in the elimination part of the programme.

It is advised that you have the bath water as hot as you can stand. Apart from the fact that warmth often alleviates arthritic pain, the heat will aid the elimination process, as will the emergence into a steamy atmosphere. It also helps in the softening of any intramuscular salt deposits which may be causing inflammation. It is suggested that the special bath is taken twice weekly as a minimum. It may be taken more often if desired, particularly if you have pain and find that the bath alleviates this for you. Do not, however, take a special bath on the fast days: the drawing and cleansing effect of the bath will also lower your blood sugar level and you may feel a little drained for a short period afterwards, although delighted with the results the following day when you will feel lighter and more mobile. The combination of the fast and the bath together can lower the blood sugar level too much and result in your becoming dizzy and weak.

There is an exercise which can be undertaken in a special bath which helps to relax the spine process. It relaxes the back muscles from top to bottom, allowing pressure on the spine to be released. Small adjustments can then take place naturally that would not otherwise have been possible. Add the sea salt, Epsom salts and ginger to 3-4 in (8-10 cm) of very hot bath water. Now lie flat on the bottom of the bath with your hands by your sides and your knees bent so the soles of your feet are flat on the bottom of the bath. Now relax and work the head from side to side until there is a release in tension, which you will hear. Now bring your knees towards your chin and hold for 30 seconds. After doing this, sit up in the bath, raise the water level and relax for 20 minutes. Finish off your bath by applying oil to the spine and affected areas. A useful tip is to put a little cotton wool with a spot of olive oil in the ears before taking the bath. This stops any of the bath additives, such as ginger, getting in the ears.

AROMATHERAPY

The massage of Rowlo Oil into the spine and affected areas strictly comes under the heading of a form of treatment called *aromatherapy* – the massage into the skin of a blend of essential oils. It is based on the knowledge that individual essential oils have particular effects on particular functions of the body. Aromatherapy is a fascinating subject and one that it is particularly pleasant to experiment with.

I have listed the ingredients of Rowlo Oil in Chapter Ten so you can mix your own. My main concern in formulating this oil was to incorporate as many of the healing properties of different oils as I possibly could into one oil. The formula is based on one that was given to me by an Indian herbalist; it is beneficial without being as greasy as most other oil combinations. If you wish to purchase some direct, write to me at the address given at the front of this book and I will give you details and send some on to you.

You do not have to restrict the use of this therapy to just after your special baths. You may practise it at any time.

If you wish to experiment further, there are many books available on this subject which describe massage techniques in detail, as also the properties of particular oils.

THE AIR YOU BREATHE

Daily deep breathing exercises will ensure that your lungs are used to the full every day. You should take any opportunity that presents itself during the day to breathe good fresh air and expand the lungs to the full to help your tissues get their much needed oxygen.

Let us now pay some attention to the air we are breathing in, as this is so important to good health and indeed to life itself.

You have no doubt been in rooms where the air feels stifling. This may not in fact be due to poor ventilation, but rather to the dearth of *negative ions* in the air.

All air contains electrically-charged particles, positive and negative ions, and it is the negative ions in the air that are important to good health. What we perceive as stuffiness is a dearth of negative ions in the air, leading to a heavy feeling which drains the energy. Negative ions are produced in nature by the ultra-violet rays of the sun, reactions in soil, in water when droplets split, and lightning. The air is so bracing in the countryside and at the sea because of an abundance of negative ions.

If you do not live in the country or at the sea, or even if you do and you have central heating, it is quite likely that the air you breathe has a depleted level of negative ions.

There is, perhaps surprisingly, something you can do about this. There are on the market today many varieties of a gadget called an ioniser. It can be found in all shapes and sizes and is available in models suitable for home, office and cars. It plugs into a socket and uses very little electricity indeed, about 2 per cent of that used by a single light bulb. Models vary in price but are available from as little as the cost of a good pair of shoes.

EXERCISE AND RELAXATION

As well as the exercise for relaxing the spine which we described under the heading of hydrotherapy, and the deep breathing exercises described above, you may like to consider walking and swimming, or more formal types of exercise such as yoga or aerobics. If you wish to try either of the latter, do so only under the guidance of an expert teacher and make sure that he knows the details of your condition. It is also worth mentioning to your doctor that you wish to take up some form of exercise.

For the more incapacitated who are following the programme, isometric exercise may be helpful. There have been many books written about these various systems of exercise, and because of this I will not go into detail about any of them. The general rule, however, is that where you feel that they are doing you good and that you are enjoying them, then continue. If they cause you pain stop them and try an easier form of exercise until such time as you have improved sufficiently to restart the ones of your choice.

Do not, under any circumstances, stretch or overwork any muscle or joint in the belief that the more pain that you have the more it is beneficial to the healing process. This is not the case. It is much more important to adopt a gentle approach on a regular basis to improve your circulation and improve your mobility.

HOMEOPATHY

Dr Hahnemann in the nineteenth century developed his theory of homeopathy into what has become today a very popular form of medicine. The British Royal Family have been ardent supporters of it for four generations.

The principle is that the body, when experiencing an illness, produces symptoms, e.g. headaches, dizzy spells, a rise in temperature, skin rashes. Hahnemann maintained that these symptoms are the manifestation of the body striving to put itself right; therefore, he suggested, a treatment should make the symptoms worse for a short period before there is an improvement in the general condition. The treatment should be a homeopathic remedy which has previously produced similar symptoms when tried out on a healthy individual.

As with herbalism, the total approach will be used by the practitioner who will take into account the patient's spiritual, mental, emotional and physical needs before assessing which remedy to prescribe. He will enquire about work and home life, eating and sleeping habits, allergies and medical history.

The method of preparing homeopathic remedies is to take the `mother tincture' and potentise the solution. Take one drop of the mother tincture and add to it nine drops of solution; this is shown as 1x. One drop of the 1x solution is then added to nine drops of the solution and this is shown as 2x. One drop of 2x is then added to nine drops of the solution and this is shown as 3x, and so on until you reach the dilution required. Thus the amount of original tincture is very small by the time it gets to the patient.

Nobody is sure how this form of treatment works, but it certainly does. When a cholera epidemic spread through Europe in the nineteenth century, patients treated by homeopathic remedies had a much higher survival rate than those treated allopathically.

ACUPUNCTURE

Acupuncture has been practised for at least 5,000 years and is currently fashionable throughout the world, the present revival being stimulated by Mao Tse Tung's 'barefoot doctors' in the 1950s.

The principle of acupuncture is to ensure that the *life force*, which flows through the body along channels called *meridians*, is maintained at its peak. This is achieved by inserting needles into various points along these channels to try to balance the flow of energy (referred to as `chi') and thereby attack the cause of disease.

More recently it has been discovered that needles stimulate the brain into releasing substances called *endorphins* which are naturally produced painkillers with a marked similarity to morphine. Now that a scientific basis has been established for this form of treatment, many hospitals are setting up pain clinics and are using acupuncture in them.

OSTEOPATHY

Osteopathy is based on the theory that mechanical faults in the structure of the body are responsible for many illnesses.

The object of the treatment is to restore movement in the spine or joint so as to free any trapped nerves and restore full blood supply to the area, thus allowing the body's own healing process to act on the disease.

The originator of the theory of osteopathy was Andrew Still, who had the unusual distinction of being both a doctor and an engineer. This led him to the conclusion that the relationship between structure and function is paramount to good health. He began to treat patients by manipulation towards the end of the nineteenth century and opened his first training school in 1892 at Kirkville, Missouri. The method quickly spread round the world with the first training school in the UK being established in 1914, just before the war. The practitioner will attempt to restore normal movement by manipulation of the joint and leverage in such a manner as to allow both the muscles and ligaments to adjust as well as the joint: a thrust action is often used, particularly in the lumbar roll, a movement often used by osteopaths in the treatment of lower back disorders.

CHIROPRACTIC

Chiropractors concentrate on the spine in their treatments in much the same way as the osteopath, by manipulating the muscles and joints to establish equilibrium by improving the circulation and freeing the nervous system.

They tend to use more aids, such as X-rays, than the osteopath, and they also use a manipulative technique of short lever, quick thrust as opposed to the long lever and rotating-type thrust of the osteopath.

The success of chiropractic has been suggested by popular support, mainly in the USA but now also in Europe, New Zealand and Canada. There are over 25,000 practitioners in the USA and they have over 40 million clients per year: sure testimony to the success of their treatments.

In undertaking chiropractic therapy, as with acupuncture and osteopathy, you would benefit more from a course of, say, ten sessions than by having sporadic bursts of treatment.

PHYSIOTHERAPY

Your doctor may well refer you to a consultant who will be able to arrange physiotherapy for you. Massage, manipulation, and applied local heat, often by electrical methods, are the physiotherapist's staple tools. He or the doctor will also recommend a series of home exercises to do between treatments. Hospital physiotherapy departments are doing magnificent work in this area but are all too often overworked, and you may be better finding a private practitioner in this field.

The therapies described above are the types of treatment that I feel you will find most useful to include in your treatment programme. You may find that one therapy helps you better than others, in which case this is the one for you. It does not mean that the others are no good, just that they do not help your particular case.

ALLOPATHIC MEDICINE

Orthodox medicine in the West is referred to as allopathic, a word which derives from the Greek words *allos* 'other' and *pathos* 'suffering'. It is the method of treating disease by the use of agents which produce effects different from the disease being treated. It thus takes the opposite standpoint from homeopathy.

The basic premise on which the doctor will be working is to reduce the pain and enable the patient to lead as normal a life as possible. He will be employing the supportive role of the physiotherapist and he will be prescribing analgesic and anti-inflammatory drugs. This is, of course, a very different approach from the one I am putting forward in this book, but it can work in parallel with a self-care treatment programme with considerable success.

CHAPTER NINE

The food guide

This Food Guide is a quick reference to the foods that you may eat when on the programme. The eight-point plan has been discussed in the previous chapter, and this has been used to calculate the percentage given to each food. To recapitulate, these factors affecting the suitability of the foods are:

- high potassium content
- low sodium content
- low sugar content
- high pantothenic acid content
- high fibre content
- the foods should be rich sources of trace elements
- the foods should contain no substances to which you, personally, react badly.

For Stages One to Three you may eat any foods below a 55% rating; for Stage Four any foods below 60%, and for Stages Five and Six, any foods below 70%.

When coming off the diet, the percentage can be increased by 5% per month and each addition to the diet should be studied for adverse reactions. If any present themselves, then that food is not for you.

Remember that, although there is no control on the quantity of any food consumed, there are borderline foods which may rate just under your percentage. You must not have too many of these in your overall diet: it should be well-balanced.

FOOD VALUES

%		%	
15	Almonds, dried	90	pie, commercial
75	Almonds, roasted, salted	75	pie, homemade
15	Apple, raw, unpeeled	85	stew, canned with vegetables
50	Apple juice, bottled	75	stew, homemade
80	Apple sauce, sweetened		Beet, beetroot
	Apricots	65	canned, regular pack
70	canned	50	cooked
20	dried	40	low sodium
75	cooked, sweetened	60	Beet greens, cooked
15	fresh		Beverages, alcoholic
75	nectar, concentrated	80	bitter beer
	Asparagus	30	lager beer
75	canned	40	mild beer
40	frozen spears, cooked	85	gin
40	green, cooked	10	table wine
40	low sodium	15	Blackberries
20	Aubergine/Egg plant, cooked	20	Blueberries
30	Avocado pear	70	Bouillon cube
		75	Bran with sugar and malt extract
70	Bacon	50	Bran flakes (40% bran)
95	Baking powder/soda	50	with raisins
15	Banana	10	Brazil nuts
15	Barley, pearled, light		Breads
15	Bass, sea	20	cracked wheat
	Beans	60	French or Vienna
50	canned	10	rye, American
5	mung	5	pumpernickel
5	sprouts	80	white, 3-4% nonfat milk solids
	Beef	20	wholemeal
95	hamburger	10	wholewheat
90	canned roast	10	Broccoli spears
85	corned	10	Brussels sprouts
85	dried		
75	lean (grilled, roasted, braised)		

%

Butter
85	salted
55	unsalted
10	Buttermilk

20	Cabbage, cooked
80	Cakes (home recipe)
85	angel food
85	chocolate with icing
45	fruit, dark
45	gingerbread
45	plain without icing
75	sponge
5	Carrots
80	canned, regular pack
45	cooked
60	low sodium
5	Cashew nuts, unsalted

Cauliflower
30	cooked
5	fresh
10	frozen, cooked

Celery
10	cooked
5	fresh
80	Chard, Swiss, cooked

Cheese, half fat
50	Caerphilly
50	Cheddar
50	Cheshire
70	cottage
70	cream
50	Danish blue
50	Edam
50	Gruyère (Swiss)
20	Parmesan

%

80	Cheese, any full fat
10	Cherries
90	canned, syrup pack
50	frozen
10	Chicken
10	Chicory
50	Chilli con carne, canned with beans
50	Chilli powder with seasonings
85	Chocolate, bitter

Clams
45	canned
35	hard, round, meat, only
30	raw, soft meat only

Coconut
75	dried, sweetened
50	fresh, shredded

Coffee
20	decaffeinated
85	instant dry powder

Corn
90	rice and wheat flakes
95	shredded
90	puffed

Corn, sweet
75	canned, whole kernel, regular pack
55	cooked
55	low sodium pack
85	Cornflakes
85	sugar-coated
70	Cornmeal/polenta or maize meal

Cowpeas
70	canned, regular pack
40	dry seeds, cooked

%		%	
60	immature, cooked	15	fresh
35	Crabmeat, canned	20	Flounder
	Crackers	20	Fruit cocktail, fresh
75	plain		Gelatine
75	soda	70	dry
40	wholewheat	75	sweetened, ready to eat
	Cranberry		
45	juice	10	Goose, flesh only
45	sauce		Grapefruit
	Cream	85	canned, sweetened
85	half and half	75	fresh
90	light coffee	75	juice
95	substitute (cream, skim milk, lactose)	20	Grapes
		20	juice, bottled
95	whipping – light		
60	Cucumbers, not peeled		Haddock
75	Custard, baked	60	fried (dipped in egg, milk, breadcrumbs)
	Dandelion	15	raw
10	coffee		Heart, beef
10	greens, cooked	80	cooked, braised
15	Dates	75	lean
75	Doughnuts, cake-type	15	Herb teas
15	Duck, flesh only	20	Herring
		50	Honey (1 teaspoonful daily only at the start of your programme – no reasonable limit when you have reached 70 in your programme)
	Eggs		
60	white		
60	whole (no more than 3 per week)		
60	yolk		
45	Endive, curly	60	Ice cream, no added salt, approximately 12% fat
10	Fats, vegetable		
	Figs	80	Jams and preserves
20	canned	80	Jellies
20	dried, uncooked		

%

10 Kale cooked, leaves with stems

75 Lamb, average of lean cuts, cooked
85 Lard
50 Lemon juice, fresh (1 daily only)
80 Lemonade, frozen, diluted
20 Lettuce
75 Lime juice, fresh or canned
75 Limeade, frozen, diluted
    Liver, cooked, fried
65 beef
65 calf
55 pork
25 Lobster, canned or cooked

25 Macaroni
70 with cheese, baked
    Margarine
75 salted
20 unsalted
    Milk
20 dry, nonfat, instant
80 evaporated, undiluted
10 goat's
20 skimmed
80 whole pasteurised
85 Milk beverages
80 chocolated flavoured, with skimmed milk
80 malted with whole milk
80 milk
30 Mineral waters
10 Molasses

%

    Mushrooms
70 canned
10 fresh
    Mustard, prepared
65 yellow
50 Mustard greens, cooked

20 Nectarine
50 Noodles

10 Oatmeal
60 cooked, salted
10 Oil, vegetable
10 Okra, cooked
    Olives
75 green
60 ripe
    Onion
15 cooked
10 fresh
    Orange
70 juice
70 peeled
10 Oyster

20 Papaya,. raw
20 Parsley
20 Parsnips, cooked
    Peach
55 canned
85 cooked with sugar
25 dried, sulphured, uncooked
10 fresh
50 frozen
85 nectar
80 Peanut butter

%	
	Peanuts
50	roasted
80	salted
	Pear
30	canned
10	fresh
95	nectar
	Peas
50	canned, regular pack
30	dry, split
30	frozen
10	green, cooked
20	low sodium pack
10	Pecans
10	Pepper, sweet, green, raw
10	Perch, ocean, Atlantic
10	Persimmon, Japanese
75	Pickles
	Pies, home recipes, wholewheat flour
75	apple
75	cherry
75	custard
90	lemon meringue
90	mince
70	Pumpkin
70	Piecrust, baked
50	Pike, walleye
	Pineapple
20	canned, unsweetened
10	fresh
10	juice, canned unsweetened
60	Pizza, cheese, home recipe
	Plums
10	canned, purple
10	fresh

%	
90	Popcorn, salted
	Pork
70	fresh, lean, roasted
70	Picnic ham, lean, simmered
	Pork, cured
80	canned, spiced or unspiced
70	ham, light cure, lean, cooked
	Potatoes
10	baked
10	boiled, unsalted
90	French fried
60	mashed with milk
75	potato chips, using vegetable oil
80	Pretzels
	Prunes
20	cooked without sugar
20	dried, uncooked
20	juice
85	Pudding, home recipe
85	bread with raisins
85	chocolate
85	cornstarch (blancmange)
85	rennin, using mix
85	rice with raisins
85	tapioca cream
20	Pumpkin, canned, unsalted
20	Radishes
20	Raisins
70	Raspberries
75	Relish (chutney)
90	Rhubarb, cooked, unsweetened
20	Rice
	Rice cereals

%

70 flakes

50 puffed, without salt

Rolls

70 commercial, plain

70 sweet

50 wholewheat

30 Rye flour, light

70 Rye wafers

Salad dressings

75 commercial mayonnaise type

75 French

60 home-cooked

65 mayonnaise

65 Thousand Island

10 Salmon, pink

55 canned

50 Sardines, Pacific, canned in tomato sauce

55 Sauerkraut

75 Sausage

75 Bologna

65 Frankfurters, raw

70 pork links, cooked

55 Scallops, bay, steamed

50 Shrimp, fresh

80 Sorbet/sherbert, orange

Soup, canned, diluted with equal part water

50 bean

70 bean with pork

75 beef bouillon

75 beef noodle

50 chicken

50 clam chowder, Manhattan type

%

50 cream soup (mushroom)

50 lentil

50 minestrone

50 onion

50 pea, green

70 tomato

80 vegetable with beef broth

20 Spaghetti

70 home recipe

70 in tomato sauce with cheese

80 with tender meatballs, canned

Spinach

50 canned, regular pack

15 cooked

10 fresh

40 low sodium

Squash

20 summer, cooked

10 winter, cooked

Strawberries

75 fresh

75 frozen

Sugar

85 brown

85 granulated

Sweet potatoes

15 baked

75 boiled, candied

75 Syrup, table blend

Tangerines

70 fresh

75 juice, canned

10 Tapioca

75 Tea

%

15 herb

Tomatoes

75 canned, low sodium

75 canned, regular pack

70 fresh

85 juice, canned, regular pack

85 ketchup, regular pack

80 Tongue, beef, braised

55 Tuna, canned in oil, solids and liquid

Turkey

15 dark

10 light

Turnip

20 cooked, diced

30 frozen

40 greens, canned, regular pack

10 Vinegar, cider

85 Waffles, home recipe

10 Walnuts

%

20 Watermelon

55 Wheat and malted barley, dry, cooked

30 Wheat, rolled, cooked

10 Wheat bran, crude

Wheat cereals

55 cooked

65 flakes

10 puffed, without salt

10 shredded, plain

Wheat flours

55 all-purpose or family cake

55 self-raising

10 wheatgerm

10 wholewheat

55 White sauce

10 Yeast, baker's

10 Yogurt, made from partially skimmed milk

CHAPTER TEN

The preparations guide

Rowlo oil

The Rowlo Oil Formula has benefited a great many of my patients. It is a unique blend of exotic, vegetable and aromatic oils that I combine to help both the arthritic joint and the blood circulation in the soft tissue. It should be applied to the affected joints as required and massaged into the spine as well as the local pain areas after the special baths.

The ingredients are as follows:
Arachis oil *Arachis hypogaea*
Cajuput oil *Melaleuca leucodendron*
Juniper berry oil *Juniperus communis*
Clove oil *Eugenia caryophyllus*
Olive oil *Olea europaea*
Avocado oil *Persea americana*
Amber oil *Pinus palustris*
Almond oil *Prunus communis*
Wintergreen oil *Gaultheria procumbens*

Obtaining supplies of Rowlo Oil or herbal preparations

If you cannot make your own, you can purchase my oil or my herbal preparations by post by writing to me at the Naturopathic Clinic – see address at the front of the book.

PARSLEY SPRINKLE

The Parsley Formula is a preparation of finely ground herbs. The ingredients are as follows:

Parsley *Petroselinum crispum*
Bearberry *Arctostaphylos uva-ursi*
Yarrow *Achillea millefolium*
Prickly ash bark *Zan thoxylum clavis herculis*
Burdock *Arctium lappa*
Poplar bark *Populus tremuloides*
Senna *Cassia angustifolia*
Alfalfa *Medicago*

CELERY COMPOUND TISANE

Rheumatic root (wild yam) *Dioscorea villosa*
Yarrow *Achillea millefolium*
Celery *Apium graveolens*
Burdock *Arctium lappa*
Chickweed *Stellaria media*
Willow bark (white willow) *Salix alba*
Alfalfa *Medicago*

Directions for use
1. Place 2 teaspoons in a small teapot.
2. Pour on 1/2 pint (300 ml) boiling water and stir.
3. Leave to stand overnight.
4. Strain. Take 1 cup after breakfast and evening meal.

Willow Bark and Meadowsweet Tablets
When the pain is acute, relief is often gained by an increased intake of willow bark with meadowsweet added.
White willow bark *Salix alba*
Meadowsweet *Filipendula ulmaria*

Kelp Tablets

Seaweeds were the first living plants on the earth and there are now over 700 recorded species. There is good reason to believe that kelp is one of the first crops to have been used by man. It was certainly used by the Chinese, the Greeks and the Romans, not only as a food, but also as a fertiliser and as a medicine. In Ireland, Wales and Japan, seaweed is a common food today.

I have found kelp to be beneficial in the treatment of underactive thyroid glands. I have mentioned earlier that our blood mimics, and therefore resembles very closely, the chemical consistency of sea water. Kelp, in absorbing the nutrients of sea water and processing them into a form that humans can use, has done a good job for us. You will not be surprised that kelp tablets are included as a supplement in your total health programme. An average analysis of kelp shows that it contains thirteen vitamins, sixty trace elements and twenty essential amino acids. Please note, particularly if you are a vegetarian, that kelp contains Vitamin B12, an ingredient that is often deficient in the vegetarian diet.

Pantothenic Acid Tablets

Each tablet contains 500 mg pantothenic acid (Vitamin B5).

Multivitamin and Mineral Formula

Although you will not be deficient in very many vitamins and minerals at any one time, by taking this formula regularly you will ensure that you lack none of the vital ingredients for making as speedy as possible a recovery. You should take two tablets daily with food.

Each tablet will provide:

Vitamins

Vitamin A (retinol)	500µg (1450 i.u.)
Vitamin D3 (cholecalciferol)	4µg (160 i.u.)
Vitamin E (dl-a tocopheryl acetate)	10mg (10 i.u.)
Vitamin C (ascorbic acid)	50mg
Vitamin B1 (thiamine HCl)	20mg

Vitamin B2 (riboflavin)	20mg
Vitamin B6 (pyridoxine HCI)	20mg
Vitamin B12 (cyanocobalamin)	4mg
Nicotinamide	20mg
Pantothenic acid	20mg
d-Biotin	150µg
Folic acid	200µg
Para-aminobenzoic acid	10mg
Choline bitartrate	10mg
Inositol	5mg

Note: 1µg = 2.907 international units (i.u.)

Minerals

Calcium (as phosphate)	126mg
Phosphorus (as phosphate)	60mg
Potassium (as phosphate)	20mg
Magnesium (as oxide)	25mg
Iron (as ferrous fumarate)	3mg
Copper (as gluconate)	100µg
Manganese (as gluconate)	2.2mg
Iodine (as kelp)	20µg
Zinc (as oxide)	1mg
Selenium (as Se yeast)	25µg

Other ingredients

Lecithin	20mg
Betaine HCI	2.2mg
dl-Methionine	2.2mg
l-Lysine HCI	1.75mg
cl-Cysteine HCI	0.25mg
Glutamic acid	4mg
Bioflavonoids complex	5mg
Dried yeast	20mg
Alfalfa	20mg

Kelp	25mg
Ginseng	20mg
Red Clover	5mg
Damiana aphrodisiaca	3mg

Aly Salt

Aly Salt is potassium chloride. It is an alternative to common sodium chloride, common table salt. It should be used sparingly on the food after cooking and not in the original food preparation. Not suitable for anybody suffering from kidney or liver disease.

Vitamin C Plus

These tablets each contain 500 mg of ascorbic acid with the addition of 50 mg of the bioflavonoid complex.

African Devil's Claw Tablets

The ingredients are sarsaparilla *(Smilax ornata)* and African devil's claw *(Harpogophytum procumbens)*.

Dandelion Herbal Compound Tisane
Yellow dock *Rumex crispus*
Burdock *Arctium lappa*
Wood sanicle *Sanicula europaea*
Buchu *Barosma betulina*
Sarsaparilla (Jamaican) *Smilax ornata*
Skullcap *Scutellaria laterifolia*
Dandelion *Taraxacum officinale*

Directions for use
1. Place 2 teaspoons in a small teapot.
2. Pour on 1/2 pint (300 ml) boiling water and stir.
3. Leave to stand overnight.
4. Strain. Take 1 cup after breakfast and evening meal.

GLOSSARY

Alterative	Helps cleanse the system of morbid matter.
Anti-bilious	Corrects the bile.
Anti-inflammatory	Reduces inflammation.
Anti-pyretic	Efficacious against fever,
Anti-rheumatic	Relieves rheumatic and arthritic conditions.
Antiseptic	Destroys micro-organisms, prevents sepsis.
Anti-spasmodic	Relieves or prevents spasm.
Carminative	Expels wind.
Demulcent	Lubricative.
Diaphoretic	Stimulates perspiration.
Diuretic	Increases the formation and discharge of urine.
Emollient	Causing warmth and moisture.
Febrifuge	Dispelling fever.
Glycoside	Any group of organic compounds found abundantly in plants which hydrolyse into sugar and other organic compounds.
Laxative	Mild purgative.
Narcotic	Relieves pain, brings on sleep and, in large doses, coma.
Nutritive	Nourishing.
Purgative	Promotes bowel action.
Resin	A semi-solid substance obtained from exudations of plants.
Saponins	Glycosides found in plants which cause water to froth.
Sedative	Soothing to the nerves.
Stomachic	Strengthens stomach and digestive organs.
Tannin	Astringent vegetable compounds.
Volatile oil	Odiferous oil obtained from plants containing a variety of chemical compounds.

Herbal Compendium

Alfalfa	*Medicago*
Almond	*Prunus communis*
Amber	*Pinus palustris*
Arachis	*Arachis hypogaea*
Avocado	*Persea americana*
Bearberry	*Arctostaphylos uva-ursi*
Bogbean	*Menyanthes trifoliata*
Buchu	*Barosma betulina*
Burdock	*Arctium lappa*
Cajuput	*Melaleuca leucodendron*
Celery	*Apium graveolens*
Chickweed	*Stellaria media*
Clove	*Eugenia caryophyllus*
Dandelion	*Taraxacum officinale*
Juniper	*Juniperus communis*
Kelp	*Laminaria spp.*
Meadowsweet	*Filipendula ulmaria*
Olive	*Olea europaea*
Parsley	*Petroselinum crispum*
Poplar bark	*Populus tremuloides*
Prickly ash bark	*Zanthoxylum clava herculis*
Rheumatic root	*Dioscorea villosa*
Sarsaparilla	*Smilax ornata*

Senna	*Cassia angustifolia*
Skullcap	*Scutellaria laterifolia*
Willow bark	*Salix alba*
Wintergreen	*Gaultheria procumbens*
Wood sanicle	*Sanicula europaea*
Yarrow	*Achillea millefolium*
Yellow dock	*Rumex crispus*

Alfalfa *Medicago*

Constituents: Source of vitamins, mineral salts, potassium, phosphorus, iron.

Action: Nutrient.

Alfalfa is a rich source of nutrients, particularly potassium, phosphorus, and iron, which are obtained by the roots of the plant which extend deep into the ground, sometimes as much as 40 feet (12 m). It has recently become a popular food supplement for people on fitness programmes and those who are convalescing.

Almond *Prunus communis*

Constituents: Fixed oil, consisting mainly of olein and a small proportion of linolein.

Action: Nutrient and demulcent.

Most people will be familiar with the almond nut, if not the oil, but we use both at some stage of the programme. The oil is one of the ingredients in Rowlo Oil which is used for the massage after the special baths and the nut will be found in the muesli.

The almond tree is mainly found in warm climates but it has always been popular in gardens in temperate climates.

The nutritive value of the nut has made it popular with naturopaths who frequently recommend that ten almonds be taken daily, chewed well.

Amber
Pinus palustris

Constituents: Properties similar to those of turpentine oil and is obtained by the distillation of certain resins or by distilling resin oil.

Amber oil *(Oleum succini)* is one of the ingredients in Rowlo Oil. It has long had a reputation for its healing properties and is included in many liniments throughout the world.

Arachis
Arachis hypogaea

Constituents: Fixed oil, proteins, starch.
Action: Nutritive, emollient.

The peanut is familiar worldwide both as a nut and as peanut butter. The oil is one of the ingredients in Rowlo Oil and has a beneficial effect on inflamed joints. On its own it is liable to go rancid, but as an ingredient in a blend of oils it lasts well.

Avocado
Persea americana

Constituents: Edible oil, the fruit has a high protein and potassium content.

Due to a highly successful cultivation and marketing programme, the avocado pear has become commonplace throughout the world and is now included in most recipe books.

I have found the oil to be of great benefit: it has a distinct cooling effect and it was for this reason that I decided some years ago to include it in the Rowlo Oil formula.

Bearberry
Arctostaphylos uva-ursi

Constituents: Tannin, acids, glycosides.
Action: Urinary antiseptic, astringent, diuretic, anti-inflammatory.

Virtually all the past and present-day herbal pharmacies would have *uva-ursi* or bearberry leaves in stock. It has certainly been used in the UK since the thirteenth century for conditions associated with inflammation of the urinary organs and its ability to act as an efficient diuretic.

It combines well with other herbs to form effective compounds.

Bogbean *Menyanthes trifoliata*
Constituents: Volatile oil, glycosides and bitters.
Action: Tonic, bitter, diuretic.

Bogbean is also referred to as buckbean and marsh trefoil. It is almost a specific herb for the treatment of arthritis and almost always appeared as part of the medicine chests in the monasteries, particularly in Germany where the plant has been held in high esteem for centuries.

I have been including this herb in my arthritis formula for some years now with excellent results and I refer to it as my bogbean compound.

Buchu *Barosma betulina*
Constituents: Volatile oil and an agent called diosphenol which has antiseptic qualities.
Action: Urinary antiseptic, diuretic, diaphoretic, anti- inflammatory.

I have found the beneficial effects of this herb to be tremendous; it has undoubted powers as a urinary antiseptic and I have achieved remarkable results by basing a formula on buchu for such conditions as cystitis, gravel and inflammation of the bladder, as well as arthritis. In fact, I had an enquiry from one of Britain's leading hospitals asking how I had successfully treated a patient of theirs with whom they had had little success. I explained that I was using a herb that was first introduced into medicine in this country in 1821 and was, for over a hundred years, the official treatment for cystitis, urethritis and catarrh of the bladder. With the advent of antibiotics it lost its popularity but not its usefulness; it is still as useful today as it was in 1821.

Burdock *Arctium lappa*
Constituents: Inulin, bitters, resin, fixed and volatile oils flavonoids, anti-bacterial substances.
Action: Mild diuretic, anti-bacterial, alterative.

Burdock was used by the herbalists in their treatment for gonorrhea before the advent of antibiotics. It has always been regarded as a strong alterative or blood cleanser and is today used in treatments for arthritis, gout, eczema an psoriasis and is often used in conjuction with slippery elm bark in treating anorexia nervosa.

Apart from its contribution to herbal medicine, burdock has two other claims to fame: the first one is the burrs which are the plant's means of disseminating itself, hence the various synonyms by which it is referred to throughout the world such as thorny burr, beggar's buttons or hoppy major. It is also one of the basic ingredients of that popular drink, dandelion and burdock.

Cajuput   *Melaleuca leucodendron*
Constituents: Volatile oil.
Action: Anti-spasmodic, diaphoretic, stimulant, antiseptic.

The cajuput tree, which is a native of the East Indies, has produced for us one of the finest volatile oils that are at present available for use in our treatment programme.

When applied externally it is a stimulant and mild counter-irritant. When taken internally, it has a highly stimulant action, producing an increased pulse rate and often profuse perspiration. In moderate doses it is used for conditions such as laryngitis, bronchitis and cystitis.

Celery   *Apium graveolens*
Constituents: Two oils, volatile and fixed.
Action: Anti-rheumatic, sedative, diuretic, urinary antiseptic, carminative.

I hold celery in high esteem and have used the seeds, prepared in various forms, as part of a treatment programme for many conditions, not just arthritis. I have found the celery aids the nervous system and helps promote a healthy sleep which is beneficial whatever your condition. Although we use the seeds in a concentrated form, please also include celery in your diet as often as possible.

Chickweed   *Stellaria media*

Constituents: Saponins.

Action: Anti-rheumatic, alterative, antiseptic, demulcent.

Chickweed spread around the world at about the same rate that the world became Westernised, and so will be familiar to most people reading this book. It has been used in herbal medicine for internal preparations and for Chickweed Ointment which is particularly useful for conditions of the skin.

Clove   *Eugenia caryophyllus*

Constituents: Volatile oil.

Action: Stimulant, carminative, aromatic.

The clove's medicinal properties are chiefly held in the volatile oil, the taste and smell of which will almost certainly be familiar to you. Externally it is best combined with other oils as it is in Rowlo Oil.

Internally it has long been used as an aid to the digestive process particularly in relieving flatulence. It may be applied directly on the gums to stop them bleeding. Recently it has started once again to be used as a natural preservative.

Dandelion   *Taraxacum officinale*

Constituents: Bitters, taraxacerin, glycosides, potassium.

Action: Anti-rheumatic, diuretic, anti-inflammatory, mild laxative.

The dandelion is a familiar plant to us all and a particularly useful one, both for its edible and medicinal properties. It gets its name from a corruption of the French name 'dent de lion' because the leaves have a jagged appearance that resembles the teeth of lions.

The leaves are used in salads and they have a slightly bitter taste when young. They are often used boiled as a substitute for spring cabbage or spinach. The plant is popular as a partner in that famous drink dandelion and burdock. The roots are roasted to form dandelion coffee - a very pleasant drink which I recommend as an excellent substitute for tea or ordinary coffee. The absence of caffeine is a bonus to anyone on a detoxification programme.

The history of dandelion as a medicinal plant goes back hundreds if not thousands of years. There are many early references in India to dandelions being most suitable for liver complaints. This is probably because the root contains a bitter substance called taraxacerin which is active against diseases of the liver.

It is also beneficial to the kidney and urinary systems and is a general stimulant to the system.

Apart from its uses in compounds for arthritis, herbalists would use it for such conditions as cholecystitis, gall stones and jaundice.

Juniper   *Juniperus communis*
Constituents: Volatile oil, bitters, organic acids.
Action: Anti-rheumatic, diuretic, anti-inflammatory, antiseptic, stomachic.

Juniper berries have been used in medicine, both herbal and allopathic, since early Greek and Roman times. The oil is chiefly used both internally for indigestion, flatulence, and diseases of the kidney and bladder, and externally, combined with other oils, as a mild stimulant for arthritic and skin conditions.

Kelp   *Laminaria spp.*
Constituents: A wide range of minerals and trace elements, the most important being iodine.
Action: Protects against infection, regulates and activates metabolism. See p79 for details of this substance.

Meadowsweet   *Filipendula (Spiraea) ulmaria*
Constituents: Essential oil with salicylic acid compounds.
Action: Anti-rheumatic, aromatic, astringent, diuretic, antacid, antiseptic.

Meadowsweet is often referred to as 'queen of the meadow' and is one of the best known wild flowers, probably due to the overall fragrance of the plant. It is unusual because the scent of the leaves is different from that of the flowers and gives much pleasure to our sense of smell.

It has been a favourite ingredient of herb beers since medieval times and there were few monasteries that did not include meadowsweet in their medicine chest, where they would use it in compounds for disorders of the stomach and bowels, and for arthritis, probably due to its salicylic content.

Olive   *Olea europaea*

Constituents: Oil, resin.

Action: Antiseptic, astringent, febrifuge, demulcent, mild laxative.

My chief interest in olive is the use of the oil in Rowlo Oil and for taking internally, combined with lemon juice, as a tonic to the liver.

You will undoubtedly be familiar with olive oil, but perhaps not aware of the process which is used for extraction. The first pressing of the fruit is achieved by crushing the olives in rough bags which are immersed in water. The oil which floats on the water is skimmed off and this oil has a slight green tint and is referred to as 'virgin' or 'first pressing'. This is available in most good shops and is the one that we want for our programme.

To obtain the second pressing of the oil, the cake is moistened and allowed to ferment: this is not the quality for us.

Parsley   *Petroselinum crispum*

Constituents: Essential oils, apiol, glycosides, Vitamin C.

Action: Aperient, diuretic, carminative.

This herb needs little in the way of description as it is widely used in cookery throughout the world. It originally became popular as a culinary herb because it is one of the richest sources of Vitamin C.

This may contribute to its diuretic action, i.e. helping the body to reduce its excess water.

It combines well with other herbs to make effective herbal compounds, particularly where there may be any congestion of the kidneys.

Poplar Bark   *Populus tremuloides*
Constituents: Salicin, populin.
Action: Anti-rheumatic, antiseptic, febrifuge, anti-inflammatory.

This was undoubtedly one of the essential herbs to be included in the medicine chest of the monasteries. It was often combined with meadowsweet for fevers, sciatica and pains of the hip.

Prickly Ash Bark   *Zanthoxylum clava hercullis*
Constituents: Volatile oil, alkaloids.
Action: Anti-rheumatic, stimulant, carminative, alterative, tonic.

The prickly ash bark is highly regarded in the USA for use in countering arthritis, skin conditions and impurities of the blood. The early settlers used the powdered bark on varicose ulcers and for cleaning old wounds. It was also made into a tonic for the system which was used in debilitating conditions of the stomach and digestive organs, such as colic and cramp. There is much interest amongst the herbal community in prickly ash due to its stimulant action which helps in circulatory conditions, such as intermittent claudication and Raynaud's syndrome.

Rheumatic Root   *Dioscorea villosa*
Constituents: Steroidal, glycosides, saponin.
Action: Anti-rheumatic, anti-inflammatory, mild diaphoretic.

There are over 150 varieties of Dioscorea and herbalists gave this one the name of rheumatic root to distinguish it from the rest. Its other name is wild yam.

It is not only an important anti-rheumatic herb, being almost a specific for arthritis, but is also particularly useful for any internal inflammation, such as cholecystitis or diverticulitis, and is also helpful in circulatory conditions such as intermittent claudication.

Its more recent claim to fame is the fact that we obtain from it the agent diosgenin which is the precursor for the manufacture of steroids and the contraceptive pill.

Sarsaparilla (Jamaican) *Smilax ornata*
Constituents: Saponins, glycosides.
Action: Anti-rheumatic, antiseptic, alterative.

Sarsaparilla is famous as a drink which is often sold alongside dandelion and burdock, each having their own distinct flavour. It is one of the strongest alteratives that we have and its powers for cleansing the blood and giving a clear skin are renowned.

It was first introduced into the UK in the sixteenth century for the treatment of syphilis and other venereal diseases, and in all probability will soon be required again as antibiotics are now starting to be non-effective in this area of disease. More recently it has been used for other chronic conditions, such as arthritis, where it is still popular to this day in herbal medicine.

Senna *Cassia angustifolia*
Constituents: Anthraquinone and derivatives.
Action: Purgative.

Senna is undoubtedly the best known of any of the herbs mentioned for this programme, its purgative action being well known for hundreds of laxative preparations.

In our programme we use the fruit of the senna, the pods, which are not quite as severe in their actions as the leaves. Senna originated in Egypt and has been cultivated in the UK since 1640.

Skullcap *Scutellaria laterifolia*
Constituents: Flavonoid glycosides, volatile oil, tannin, bitters.
Action: Sedative, anti-spasmodic.

Before stronger synthetic sedatives came onto the market, skullcap was considered to be almost a specific for the convulsive twitchings of St Vitus' Dance.

It still has a tremendous following amongst insomniacs as a pleasant way of inducing sleep without any of the unpleasant side effects of synthetic drugs.

The anti-spasmodic effect of skullcap has ensured its place in the folklore of Europe and the USA for its ability to cure hiccups.

Willow Bark   *Salix alba*

Constituents: Tannin, salicin.
Action: Anti-rheumatic, anti-inflammatory, antiseptic, analgesic, anti-pyretic.

Willow bark is an excellent source of salicin which is closely related to aspirin (which is in fact acetylsalicylic acid). It is probably for this reason, and the tannin content, that this herb has gained its high reputation.

In the treatment programmes, this herb is combined with meadowsweet.

Wintergreen   *Gaultheria procumbens*

Constituents: Volatile oil containing methyl salicylate.
Action: Stimulant, astringent, aromatic.

We are particularly interested in wintergreen for its volatile oil content which is one of the ingredients in Rowlo Oil. It has a particularly beneficial effect when combined with other oils and applied externally to the affected areas. It is also a useful oil for sportsmen to apply to the muscles to avoid mid-game cramp and maintain supple muscles.

Wood Sanicle   *Sanicula europaea*

Constituents: Tannin, bitters.
Action: Astringent, alterative, anti-inflammatory.

The origin of the name sanicle is the Latin word 'sano', 'heal or cure'.

In the Middle Ages, it gained a high reputation for treating conditions of the blood, being said to cleanse the body of morbid material, leaving the blood healthier and in better condition. This is just right for the arthritis programme where detoxification is the main theme.

It is often combined with other herbs rather than used on its own.

Yarrow   *Achillea millefolium*
Constituents: Volatile oil, glyco-alkaloid, tannin.
Action: Diuretic, diaphoretic, anti-pyretic, astringent, hypotensive.

Yarrow has a wonderful reputation throughout the world of herbal medicine for its ability to combine well with other herbs. On its own it is almost a specific for disorders of the circulatory system and arthritic conditions.

It has long been a favourite herb of mine, particularly when combined with rutin.

Yellow Dock   *Rumex crispus*
Constituents: Glycosides, tannin.
Action: Laxative, alterative, anti-rheumatic.

Yellow dock contains the same glycoside (hydroxy-anthraquinone) as senna which accounts for its laxative powers, but it also contains other agents which make the overall effect of this herb not as searching as senna. It is a useful blood purifying agent and makes an excellent member of a compound to treat arthritis and skin diseases.